Chiropractic Speaks Out

A REPLY TO MEDICAL PROPAGANDA, BIGOTRY AND IGNORANCE

Chiropractic Speaks Out

A REPLY TO MEDICAL PROPAGANDA, BIGOTRY AND IGNORANCE

BY

Chester A. Wilk, D.C.

Published by
WILK PUBLISHING CO.
P.O. Box 320, Park Ridge, Illinois 60068

CHIROPRACTIC SPEAKS OUT: A REPLY TO MEDICAL PROPAGANDA, BIGOTRY AND IGNORANCE

First Revised Edition, 1976

Library of Congress Catalog Card Number: 73-82888

Manufactured in the United States of America

Dedicated to my wife, ARDITH, for her understanding and patience during the preparation of this manuscript; to my three daughters, KIM, CATHY and CINDY; and to the millions of people everywhere who deserve the best possible health care.

"Honor a physician with the honor due unto him, for the uses which ye may have of him: for the Lord hath created him."

Apocrypha, Ecclesiasticus 38:1

Preface

SINCE chiropractic was founded in 1895, it has been the subject of great controversy. On one side are many persons and organizations praising the profession. On the other is organized medicine, which attacks chiropractic and labels it a cult not deserving of existence as a healing art.

Organized medicine has originated or supported many statements attacking chiropractic. The most common ones are included in this book to help eliminate the confusion about chiropractic, and to bring it into perspective. These will serve also as examples of organized medicine's propaganda, bigotry, monopoly, ignorance and plagiarism.

For a long time, organized medicine has enjoyed prestige and relative immunity from public criticism. In recent years, however, its well-publicized battles with Medicare, Congress, labor, the news media, senior citizen organizations, moderate and liberal medical physicians, and independent healing professions have reduced its public image to its lowest level in history. People are now questioning the sincerity of organized medicine's concern for the welfare of the public.

The time has come for chiropractic to speak out. The time has also come for the printing of this book, which was written to show that organized medicine is placing a vicious and cruel restraint upon the public by dissuading many people from chiropractic care, a care that unquestionably has eliminated needless suffering of countless people who have failed to get help through medicine. Chiropractic is not a cure-all, but neither is medicine.

It is, therefore, the purpose of this book to help bring light into the shadows of ignorance and prejudice in healing.

Acknowledgments

To those who may cast stones, let them come out of their glass houses and throw them at my door. To those who may spread laurels, let them do so at many doors. This book is the end product of the labors of many.

I am indebted to Dr. Louis O. Gearhart, Dr. Andries M. Kleynhans, Dr. Lawrence Levin, Dr. J. F. McAndrews, John "Tritt" Willisson, L. Ward Zilliox, and Richard Zwolinski. Their wisdom, knowledge and unselfish contributions were indispensable in the preparation of this manuscript.

I am grateful to the American Chiropractic Association and the International Chiropractors Association for their assistance and cooperation.

Finally, I am indebted to Michael Murphy and Dr. Martin "Marty" Stone for their help in editing the manuscript.

Contents

Introduction

WHEN my grandfather, Dr. Daniel David Palmer, discovered the principle of chiropractic in 1895, he intuitively knew of the many challenges lying ahead for the new natural healing science of chiropractic. In his writings, "D.D.," as he was affectionately known, occasionally made reference to his long hours of study, which led to his original chiropractic philosophy and the first adjustment. He felt it necessary to have a firm foundation for his healing science so it would thrive throughout the world.

Chiropractic has grown into mankind's largest natural healing art. The road has had many obstacles confronting the young science of health. Because of D.D.'s and his son, B.J.'s, determined efforts as they wrested out the basic truths of chiropractic, the profession has survived to bring great comfort and health to millions of people all over the world.

CHIROPRACTIC SPEAKS OUT will appeal to the inquisitive and searching mind. In its pages, you will read of the history of the profession and learn of the difficulties encountered during its nearly eight decades of existence. It is interesting and appealing to laymen and chiropractors alike.

DAVID D. PALMER, D.C.

CHAPTER I

History of Manipulation

EARLY MANIPULATION

THE ORIGIN of tissue manipulation is lost in antiquity but records indicate that it has existed throughout the world since the beginning of recorded time.

Some of the earliest indications of tissue manipulation is demonstrated by the ancient Chinese Kong Fou Document written about 2700 B.C. which was brought to the western world by missionaries.

A Greek papyrus dating back to at least 1500 B.C. gave instructions on the maneuvering of the lower extremities in the treatment of low back conditions.

Ancient American Indian hieroglyphics demonstrated "backwalking" in which patients would have their backs manipulated by the feet of other persons. Also, the early natives of the Polynesian Islands had children walk on the backs of ailing adults.

Some Indian tribes which used manipulative therapy were the Sioux, Winnebago and Creek Indians of North America as well as the Aztec, Toltec, Tarascan, Zoltec and Mayan Indians of Mexico and Central America. The sophisticated Inca Indians of South America were also known to practice manipulative methods.

Tissue manipulation also was practiced by the ancient Japanese, Indians of Asia, as well as the Egyptians, Babylonians, Syrians, Hindus and Tibetans.

Manipulative therapy has been practiced by the natives of Tahiti for centuries. Documentation of this can be found in the ship's log of Capt. James Cook, famous English navigator, explorer and cartographer of the late 1700s. His credits and honors are many, but he is probably best known for his rediscovery of the Hawaiian Islands.

The magnitude of his responsibilities, compounded by concern for his crew and his leaky and badly refitted ships, adversely affected his health. His digestion was disturbed, and he was developing crippling rheumatism which was aggravated by damp and leaky living quarters. Although he was a humane man making friends wherever he went, his health and the pressures of his job had an adverse effect on his daily activities. When he landed in Tahiti, he told a chief of the natives of his rheumatic pains. "We'll fix that," said the chief.

Twelve large, muscular women boarded a canoe and were paddled out ceremoniously to Capt. Cook's ship. Once on board they headed for the captain's quarters. Surrounding him, they laid a mattress and blankets on the floor of his cabin. "Lie!" they said. Since he didn't seem to have much of a choice, Cook obliged them. Promptly, they swarmed all over him, pummeling and squeezing him mercilessly with strong agile hands until his joints crackled and his flesh felt like abused blubber. After 15 minutes of these manipulations, they released Capt. Cook. To his amazement, he felt immensely better. "More?" asked the ladies. Indeed, agreed the captain. After three more such treatments his pains vanished.

The ancient "bonesetters" of England and Europe used manipulative techniques for centuries, many acquiring great fame as healers. The famous surgeon, Sir James Paget, wrote in the *British Medical Journal* January 5, 1865, an article entitled, "Cases That Bonesetters Cure." He reflected on the economic threat these bonesetters were to medical doctors when he wrote, "Few of you are likely to practice without a bonesetter for a rival; and if he can cure a case which you have failed to cure, his fortune may be made and yours marred. Learn then to imitate what is good and avoid what is bad in the practice of bonesetters."

Sir John Callie, M.D. also wrote of the bonesetters: "General practitioners as a rule know little or nothing of bonesetting. The medical profession is discredited in this way. Some bonesetters get more and more expert in manipulative dexterity in the same way as some of us play games or the violin better than others. In spite of the profession's knowledge of anatomy, physiology and pathology, the unqualified gets the credit because he cures."

Exaggerated claims of cures by the early manipulators (bonesetters, osteopaths, chiropractors) alienated the orthodox medical community. Bitterness between orthodox medicine and the manipulators ensued.

Gradually, the more contemporary manipulators became more clinically and scientifically oriented, and less prone to rash claims. But unpleasant memories remained, and many physicians retained closed minds to any scientific advances made by the manipulators. Other medical physicians, though realizing the merit of manipulation, selfishly rejected it behind the guise of "scientific unacceptability." In spite of these tribulations, man continued to advance to spinal manipulation because of apparent results. The advancement, coming from every corner of this earth for more than 5,000 years, is not without reason. As long as man walks this earth, he will continue to gravitate toward it. Manipulation with results has passed the test of time.

HIPPOCRATES

Hippocrates, the celebrated Greek physician who lived from 460 to 357 B.C., recognized the importance of spinal manipulation. A prolific writer, he has written at least 70 books on healing, including, *Manipulation and Importance to Good Health* and *On Setting Joints by Leverage*. Emphasizing the importance of the spine, he said, "Get knowledge of the spine, for this is the requisite for many diseases."

He was the first to add science to medicine and to separate the practice of medicine from religion, magic, superstition and omens. He strongly emphasized the healing power of nature and the natural recuperative power of the body. He stressed the importance of rest, fresh air, sunlight, proper diet, exercise in moderation, cleanliness, tissue manipulation, and minimum usage of drugs.

The medical profession adopted Hippocrates as the "Father of Medicine" and his Hippocratic Oath is publicly administered to medical students upon graduation from most medical schools.

CLAUDIUS GALEN

Claudius Galen was a famous Greek physician living from 130 to 200 A.D. He is considered the greatest anatomist and physiologist of classical time. He dissected monkeys, sheep, dogs, pigs, oxen, and bears, and in this manner gained much valuable knowledge which was applicable to human anatomy. However, lacking human bodies to dissect, he reached many false conclusions about human anatomy which were to remain undisputed for 1,400 years. A prolific author, he wrote 500 books during his lifetime.

Galen was given the title, "Prince of Physicians" after he corrected a paralysis of the right hand of Eudemus, a prominent Roman scholar. He did so by treating the patient's neck, apparently adjusting the neck vertebrae. Galen's fame spread throughout Rome and he was called "the wonder worker." Finally the Roman Emperor Aurelius proclaimed, "There is but one physician—Galen!"

Galen, like Hippocrates, also recognized the importance of

the nervous system when he said, "Look to the nervous system as the key to maximum health."

THE BIBLE

The Book of Esther, written in 474 B.C., refers to appropriate food, and "massage procedures" with myrrh and balsam oils. The importance of massage procedures for maximum health and beauty are emphasized in this book.

The importance of cleanliness in both physical and moral well-being is mentioned over 200 times in the Bible. These stress the cleanliness of water, food, clothing, bathing and proper latrine methods. The Book of Leviticus stresses measures with leprosy and venereal disease, and cautions against omens and magic.

Current medical literature will tell you that medical science has increased the longevity of people in recent years. The credibility of that statement is challenged by the fact that the life expectancy during Biblical times is given in the Bible as "three score and ten"—which is 70 years of age. Thus people are not living longer today than they did in the Holy Land 2,000 years ago. However, the people of Biblical times observed proper hygienic and sanitary measures.

With the fall of the Roman Empire and through the dark ages that followed, proper hygiene and sanitation became nonexistent. Great masses of people died and, of course, longevity took a severe drop, too.

Ironically, the principles of proper hygiene and sanitation as taught in the Bible, were ignored until the turn of this century. These basic principles were rejected and violated by the physicians, many of whom would condemn anyone who tried to tell them otherwise.

Thus it was not any miracle pill which restored our longevity back to the Biblical days, but proper public health and sanitation measures, the kind originally opposed by medicine. Credit must be given where credit is due.

THE DARK AGES

The death of Galen, the Roman conquest of Greece, and finally, the fall of the Roman Empire to the Barbarians in 476 A.D. plunged mankind's 2,000 years of accumulated knowledge and civilization virtually into oblivion.

The prevention and treatment of disease also took a grave step backwards. Early medicine was replaced with omens, superstitions, magic potions, witchcraft and the boiling of witches instead of water. Sanitation became nonexistent, and ignorance, pestilence and filth prevailed while logic and science took a back seat.

The physicians of the Middle Ages did not perform surgery, considered it beneath their dignity, and felt it belonged to the executioner or the barber. Physicians were accused of spreading epidemics so that they could become wealthy treating the sick. Persons accused of spreading diseases often were mercilessly tortured, their bodies were mutilated and dismembered, and they were burned to death.

Pregnant women in difficult labor were scorned and left to die or be butchered by a vagabond surgeon or hog-gelder. Men were not allowed to deliver babies. Dr. Wertt of Hamburg in 1522 put on the dress of a woman to study a case of a woman in labor. As a punishment for his audacity he was burned to death.

Although ancient Rome had paved streets 2,000 years ago, Paris had no paved streets until the 11th century and London none until the 16th century.

The Greeks of 1800 B.C. had more sophisticated ventilation, drainage, and latrine habits than the rest of the civilized world acquired in another 3,600 years—up to 170 years or so ago, as a matter of fact. Human excreta was dumped on the unpaved streets of cities and villages. It caused foul odors, breeding of flies and diseases which subsequently killed millions.

Tissue manipulation also suffered a setback. Some manipulators associated themselves with recitals of incantations during their manipulations. The vertebral "pop" so well known to chiropractic patients was said to be the "demons" being driven from the patients.

The Medico-Chemical School of healing came into vogue in the 16th century. Practitioners of this school of thought believed in fighting "evil sickness" with evil brews. The brews to fight evil consisted of snakes, or the appendages of rats, bats, toads and whatever wicked potion was handy. Of course, the more unpleasant it sounded, the better. Thus the poor, worthless, or even dangerous medications of that era were replaced with even worse ones.

The insane were chained in madhouses or jails; badly fed and naked, they would lie in their own excreta until they died of disease, neglect and exposure. Their only treatment was an occasional flogging when their cries became annoying. Incredibly, this was common practice until the latter part of the 19th century.

Surgery was not considered a part of medicine. Bloodletting, practiced by the early surgeons and barbers, was believed to be a means of reducing what they felt was an excessive supply of blood. Bloodletters would advertize their service by smearing fresh blood on poles in front of their place of business, which would signify a bandage around a bleeding white arm. Of course, the fresher and brighter the blood on the pole, the better the barber-surgeon. Since blood would darken and discolor, one ingenious barber-surgeon decided to outdo his rivals by using bright red paint. The idea caught on and we had the birth of the red-striped barber pole, the symbol of a barber shop today. In parts of Europe today the barber pole is set in a basin similar to the kind used for bloodletting. In this country, as early as the 1930s, barbers practiced cupping, or the application of suction cups on the back of a person for the purpose of drawing blood to the surface. This, they believed, would relieve muscular aches, pains and colds.

Joseph Smith, the founder of the Mormon Church, was one of the most famous "magnetic" healers of his time. Actually, he admitted using great manual force during his healings. He wrote that some of the bones of people he contacted made the noise of a "crushed basket." Thus, it becomes likely that Smith was one of the great spinal manipulators of his era.

Revival of the principles of Hippocrates began in the 16th century during the renaissance of European civilization. Through the turbulent lives of Paracelsus, Servetus, Vesalius, Harvey, Semmelweis, Bodington, Lister, Pasteur, Nightingale, Kenny, Palmer and others came a gradual transition to greater knowledge within the healing professions about the prevention and treatment of diseases.* As we review the relatively sophisticated 1970s, it is difficult to imagine the state of ignorance which existed in the healing profession just a few years ago, but the biographies of the above mentioned people speak for themselves. It is even more difficult to imagine a world today without their great contributions.

CHAPTER II

An Introduction to Chiropractic

CHIROPRACTIC ORIGIN AND GROWTH

CHIROPRACTIC was founded by Dr. Daniel David Palmer in 1895. He wrote in his first book, "I am not the first person to replace vertebrae, but I do claim to be the first to replace displaced vertebrae by using the spinous and transverse processes as levers . . . and to develop the philosophy and science of chiropractic." He also wrote in the same book, ". . . too much or not enough nerve energy is disease." The true genius of Dr. Palmer is clearly demonstrated by recent medical research which supports the concept of nerve facilitation and inhibition, and its effect upon normal health and body function.

A classic experiment occurred when Dr. Palmer had the opportunity to observe the deafness of a janitor who could not hear the ticking of a clock or the sound of wagon wheels on the cobblestone street, although he was able to hear well enough while carrying on a conversation.

The janitor advised Dr. Palmer that 17 years earlier he was in a stooped and cramped position when he felt something "give" in his back. Ever since, he had suffered the hearing defect. Dr. Palmer remembered the teaching of his old acquaintance, Dr. Jim Atkinson, who had tried unsuccessfully to promulgate spinal manipulation. Dr. Palmer then palpated the upper thoracic area where the janitor indicated his sensation had taken place, and made a vertebral adjustment. The janitor then observed that his hearing improved.

Contemporary medical research supporting Dr. Palmer's early discovery includes audiometric studies of patients, before and after spinal treatments. Extensive bibliographies of documented cases, have been reported in Vol. 24 of the medical publication, *Clinical Orthopedics.*

Thus, Dr. Daniel David Palmer's clinical results with a janitor by the name of Harvey Lillard helped bring about the birth of the art and science of chiropractic.

The word chiropractic was derived from the Greek words "cheir" and "praktikas" meaning "done by hand." Chiropractic was given a sophistication; a formal educational program was evolved; requirements by the schools were developed; and state governing laws were established. Spinal adjusting was removed from the father-to-son level so that knowledge of it could accumulate and grow. Thus, chiropractic grew and became the largest drugless healing profession in the world.

PROFESSIONAL UNITY

During its growth chiropractic has felt the "growing pains" typical of all healing professions. Although differences of opinion have existed, and still do, the profession has consistently agreed on the basic principle of chiropractic. The similarity can be easily demonstrated. The American Chiropractic Association (ACA) says: "Chiropractic is based on the premise that the relationship between structure and function in the human body is a significant health factor and that such relationships between the spinal column and the nervous system are the most significant, since the normal transmission and expression of nerve energy are essential to the restoration and maintenance of health."

The American Chiropractic Association defines chiropractic in accordance with the foregoing principle as follows: "Chiropractic is that science and art which utilizes the inherent recuperative powers of the body and the relationship between the musculo-skeletal structures and functions of the body, particularly of the spinal column and the nervous system, in the restoration and maintenance of health."

In the same vein the International Chiropractors Association (ICA) says: "Chiropractic is that science and art which utilizes the inherent recuperative powers of the body, and deals with the relationship between the nervous system and the spinal column, including its immediate articulations, and the role of this relationship in the restoration and maintenance of health."

Critics have attempted to exaggerate the difference within chiropractic and confuse this issue in an effort to undermine the public's confidence in chiropractic. But this becomes unrealistic if one considers differences typical of all professional groups, especially medicine. Furthermore, chiropractors all generally agree on the basic principle of chiropractic. The other differences are secondary, but can provide a basis for exchange of ideas, research and growth of chiropractic. The two national chiropractic organizations submitted a unified joint statement in a "white paper" dated May, 1969. The joint statement concerned chiropractic and the need for including it in Medicare. The chiropractic profession has also testified before House and Senate committees in unified joint statements also regarding chiropractic and Medicare, both positive actions of unity. Both national organizations firmly agree that chiropractic must remain a separate and distinct healing profession. They also agree that drugs and surgery have a definite merit, but do not belong within the scope of chiropractic's therapy.

PRINCIPLE AND SCOPE OF CHIROPRACTIC

Doctors of chiropractic employ a method of healing which gives particular attention to the structural and neurological aspects of the body, particularly the spine, in the prevention and treatment of human ailments. Chiropractors begin examinations by taking histories and utilizing many well known standard diagnostic techniques and instruments. Various laboratory tests and x-rays may be used to complete an examination.

Although chiropractors are generally concerned with a variety of approaches to healing, they are commonly identified as using spinal adjustments for the restoration of health. Depending on regulations various states may impose, and the chiropractor's judgment, they also may employ other approaches such as corrective exercises, physical therapeutic modalities, regulation of diet, food supplementation, restriction of activities, and advise rest and proper hygiene. In fact, they may utilize any therapeutic measures other than drugs or surgery. Though laws may vary with different states as to what chiropractors may utilize in their therapy, the chiropractic adjustment is recognized in all states where chiropractic is licensed.

ADJUSTING SUBLUXATIONS

The human spinal column has 24 presacral bony segments which are called vertebrae and, except for the top segment, are separated by elastic discs. Between the vertebrae are openings called intervertebral foramina, which are created by the articulation of the vertebrae above and below it. Exiting from these intervertebral foramina are nerves which control many body functions, including the digestive, endocrine, vascular or circulatory, muscular, and respiratory or pulmonary systems. These nerves may convey the sensation of pain, and control muscle and visceral activity.

Since the vertebrae are movable, they can become limited within their normal range of movement and may become attended by muscle spasm, tight ligaments, pain, ischemia, and decreased motion of the joints with adverse influence on nerve function. Chiropractors commonly refer to this as a vertebral subluxation.

Medical and chiropractic authorities alike have demonstrated, through scientific research and clinical studies, the existence of subluxations. Cineroentgenology (x-ray movies) of the spine taken with special x-ray equipment also have demonstrated their existence.

Dr. James P. Warbasse, former chief surgeon of the German Hospital, and attending surgeon at Methodist Episcopal Hospital in Brooklyn, said, "Subluxations of vertebrae occur in all parts of the spine and in all degrees. When the dislocation is so slight as not to affect the spinal cord, it will still produce disturbances in the spinal nerves, passing off through the spinal foramina . . ."

A chiropractor may adjust the vertebrae in an effort to remove this nerve disturbance, thereby permitting the body to function in a better state of health.

CHIROPRACTIC AND DISEASE

Contrary to AMA supported literature, modern chiropractic does not adhere to the "single cause—single cure theory" in the treatment of human ailments. Nor does it reject the pathogenicity of bacteria, viruses and other microorganisms. Bacteriology is a part of the curriculum of all chiropractic colleges.

A confusion may arise from the differentiation between *exciting* and *predisposing* causes of disease. Microorganisms are the exciting factors, causing the disease. Lowered tissue resistance is a predisposing factor, permitting the disease to overtake the body. Thus, when chiropractic refers to vertebral subluxations with altered nerve energy as causing lowered tissue resistance, a predisposing cause of disease is the intended meaning.

Medical textbooks frequently discuss predisposing and exciting causes of disease. The real issue is not one of differences between chiropractic and medicine on these causes, but rather of distortion and confusion in the matter of what chiropractic really believes and what the medical profession says chiropractic believes.

Dr. A. E. Homewood, dean of the Canadian Memorial Chiropractic College, wrote a paper on chiropractic's view on the cause of disease, which was published in the *University of Toronto Medical Journal.* He wrote: "Palmer was not unmindful of the detrimental effects of pathogenic microorganisms, the psychosomatic background of many conditions, the ill effects of unsanitary conditions, the adverse influence of faulty diet, the stress of occupation, the irritation of chemicals taken into the body either through the digestive or respiratory systems, and, of course, the evils of mechanical trauma. . . . in many areas of his book stressed the diversity of cause. . . . Unfortunately for the health of the public, allopathic medicine became enamoured with microorganisms and viruses and the chiropractic profession lost sight of the basic causes of disease, mechanical, chemical and mental stress. . . . that health does not come merely by taking medicine or structural adjustments, that the individual must obey the laws of Nature to maintain or regain health. Thus the present day patient expects to take his treatment, pay his bill, and be rewarded with health, which he will immediately begin to destroy by the manner in which he continues to live. He does not expect his doctor to insist upon good posture, proper nutrition, exercise, fresh air, correct use of his body and mind at work and play."

CHIROPRACTIC TREATS THE PATIENT

In references to the chiropractic treatment of different ailments, it should be pointed out that chiropractic treatments are not intended to be interpreted in the usual sense. Chiropractors actually do not treat diseases, they treat the patient in an attempt to help return his body to a normal state of function, thereby permitting the body to overcome the ailments.

The human body has a natural capacity to be healthy and chiropractic recognized this fact by "helping the body help itself" through its mode of treatment. The words of the prominent American medical physician, Dr. Oliver Wendell Holmes, clearly illustrated the point when he said, "Nature cures, but the doctor pockets the fee."

WHEN TO VISIT A CHIROPRACTOR

In 1962 Batten and Associates, Inc., conducted a national survey and statistical study of chiropractic. Over 6,000 chiropractors from every state in the United States and Canada participated.

Statistics were obtained in a study of chiropractic patients, and a report of their most common ailments prepared.

Another group of statistics was compiled to determine which patients showed the best results under chiropractic care. Surprisingly enough, and with only minor variations, the patients showing "best results" closely paralleled the patients "most frequently treated" by the chiropractors.

It must not be implied from the following list of ailments that chiropractic contends to have a cure-all method of healing. Dr. Alan Stoddard, a prominent doctor of physical medicine and author of the book *Manual of Osteopathic Practice*, illustrated the role of spinal manipulation in healing when he wrote: "To claim that mechanical lesions are the only etiological factors in disease is, of course, ludicrous. They are rarely if ever totally responsible, but they cannot or should not be discounted in any disease. The degree of significance of mechanical factors varies from disease to disease and from patient to patient. The mechanical component in the etiology of syphilis is negligible (if we ignore the mechanism of transmission!) but in the etiology of sciatica it is all important; and in some cases of constipation, dysmenorrhea, or asthma the mechanical factor may be so important that until the mechanics are put right the symptoms will persist.

"When all medical investigations are negative in patients in whom symptoms persist there is frequently a mechanical or structural basis for those symptoms even though the linkage seems tenuous. It is unwise to label such patients as neurotic until the mechanics of the spine have been properly assessed."

Here is a list of the most common ailments found in patients treated by chiropractors. The ailments, listed in a descending order of frequency, are:

- Headache
- Lumbosacral strain or sprain.
- Low back disorders
  - Low back syndrome
  - Lumbago
- Cervical syndrome
  - Cervical subluxations
  - (neck) head
- Spinal subluxations
  - Back injuries
  - Spinal distortion
  - Subluxations
- Sacroiliac strains
- Gastrointestinal
  - Digestive disorders
  - Nutritional deficiency
  - Stomach disorders
- Nervous disorders
  - Nervous tension
  - Neurasthenia
- Neuritis
- Arthritis
- Sciatica
- Extremity trauma (sprains)
  - Ankle
  - Knee
  - Orthopedic conditions
  - Shoulder
- Bursitis
- Respiratory conditions
- Musculoskeletal conditions
  - Neuromuscular
- Sprains
- Common Cold
- Sinusitis
- Trauma
- Dorsal conditions
  - Thoracic
- Strains
- Cardiovascular conditions
  - Heart trouble
- Hypertension
  - High blood pressure
- Emotional problems
- Neurological diseases
- Cerebrospinal conditions
- Bronchial Asthma
- Torticollis
- Whiplash injuries
- Migraine
- Rheumatism

Each of the above patient's conditions were scored by the number of times any chiropractor would list them as ailments of one of his "top-three" patients treated. There were patients with other conditions listed in this category by Batten and Associates, Inc., but they are deleted here because they received less than 100 votes total out of over 18,000 votes cast. Finally, after the patient's condition is corrected through chiropractic care, the chiropractor may recommend periodic spinal "tune-ups" as preventive maintenance care. Many patients receiving regular chiropractic adjustments benefit with better health and vitality.

HOW TO SELECT YOUR PERSONAL CHIROPRACTOR

Selecting your personal chiropractor is an important decision and should be done with utmost care and consideration.

Patient referral is a common and useful means of finding a chiropractor, but it should be based on the doctor's ability, his thoroughness in conducting an history and examination, his concern for the patient, his willingness to take time to answer the patient's questions, and the intelligence of his answers. Selecting a doctor primarily on his bedside manners does not assure you a good choice. A doctor's professional competency is not measured by his professional image alone, nor is the doctor with crude bedside manners necessarily less competent.

A chiropractor should be a member of his state and national chiropractic associations. These organizations strive to advance the quality of chiropractic care and protect it from the hostile and politically oriented organized medicine which tries to legislate it out of existence. Choose a chiropractor who, through his membership in these organizations, supports your right to receive chiropractic health care.

Local chiropractic societies can be helpful in giving you information on a chiropractor before you make an appointment with him. Several states have more than one chiropractic organization, but it does not matter which one a chiropractor belongs to, as long as he or she is a member.

Doctors that rely upon flamboyant advertising should be avoided since they are in violation of their professional code of ethics.

It must be concluded that there is no absolute formula that you can rely upon in choosing a chiropractor. The same, of course, holds true for any kind of doctor. However, following the above suggestions should enhance your chances of making a good selection.

CHAPTER III

Chiropractic Recognition and Validity

CHIROPRACTIC IS RECOGNIZED

AMONG the most common questions asked are, "Why doesn't medicine recognize chiropractic?" or "Why isn't chiropractic recognized?" One point must be made very clear at this time: CHIROPRACTIC IS RECOGNIZED. It is a licensed profession in 49 states, the District of Columbia, and Puerto Rico. Legislators have defended chiropractic's right to be licensed.

A good example of the courts supporting chiropractic licensing was demonstrated in the Illinois case in 1917 of *People v. Love*, 298 Illinois 304: "It is not the province of the courts to extol or belittle chiropractic, osteopathy or medicine or surgery. They are now established as useful professions, and as time has progressed it has been thoroughly demonstrated that all of them have accomplished, and all are daily accomplishing, the relief and cure of human ailments . . . Constantly comes proof before the courts that chiropractic does enable the chiropractor to relieve and cure many of the ailments of human beings, and that the practice of this science is in no way deleterious to the human body. That is the proof of this record."

Chiropractic is the largest, drugless healing profession in the world. It is officially classified with dentistry, medicine and osteopathy as one of four major healing professions. The classification was made by the Office of the President, U.S. Bureau of Budget, Washington, D.C.

The United States Office of Education has attested to the validity of the degree of doctor of chiropractic on page 169 of its current edition of *Academic Degrees.*

Medicare and Medicaid recognizes the services of chiropractic. Most private insurance companies recognize and pay claims for chiropractic care because of favorable statistics concerning patient improvement. They certainly would not voluntarily pay claims for something not proven valid.

Workmen's compensation boards in 49 states pay chiropractic claims. Furthermore, a national survey of workmen's compensation cases in 44 states and Canada compared medicine and chiropractic for the treatment of back conditions. The result of this survey was reported in the *Canada Foundry Journal* in 1956. It concluded: "Spinal injuries are one of the commonest causes of time-loss and pay-loss in industry. This is especially true, of course, in heavy industry. . . . The results of this survey proved conclusively that chiropractic care of low back injuries has no equal and can be of tremendous benefit in reducing the lost man hours and lost wages suffered by those afflicted with this painful condition."

In 1960, a study was made of workmen's compensation records from the state of Florida. It was entitled, *A Survey and Analysis of the Treatment of the Sprain and Strain Injuries of the Back and Neck in Industrial Cases.* The study covered 19,666 cases studied by the First Research Corporation, a nationally recognized independent research firm. The average patient under chiropractic care returned to work in three days, while the patients under medical care took nine days and the compensation costs were 311 per cent higher. Such statistics certainly serve to validate the effectiveness of chiropractic.

Other studies of state workmen's compensation cases were

made in Colorado, Iowa, Oregon, Kansas and Minnesota. In these studies the results of chiropractic and medical treatment for back conditions were compared which provided dramatic evidcncc of chiropractic's effectiveness.

In personal injury cases, courts recognize the expertise of doctors of chiropractic in the same way as they accept the testimony of doctors of medicine, podiatry or osteopathy. Furthermore, as we will see later in the book, chiropractic can often do more to help persons with these injuries than any other kind of health care.

The value of chiropractic has been demonstrated by chiropractic research and clinical studies, and by the research and clinical studies of prominent medical physicians who have reported their findings in leading medical journals throughout the world; through medical symposia and seminars; and by formation of medical societies which have stressed the manipulative approach to healing.

Many senior citizen, labor, veteran, civil service, ethnic and fraternal organizations have adopted resolutions commending the chiropractic profession.

Fifty million patients, including millions of new ones each year, seek the services of chiropractors. These patients represent all walks of life.

As we discuss these and other facts in more detail in subsequent chapters, the validity of chiropractic will become self evident as an overwhelming case will unfold for it—one that should remove any doubt from the mind of the most critical observer.

CHAPTER IV

Confusion About Chiropractic

CONFUSION about the validity of chiropractic often arises from the hostile propaganda which has been supported by organized medicine. Actually, it is not medicine's province to "recognize" chiropractic any more than it would be chiropractic's province to "recognize" medicine. This could be compared to asking a Democrat or Republican which party has the better solution for running government. Organized medicine has clearly demonstrated its prejudice with its record of attack or attempted monopoly of optometry, osteopathy, homeopathy, chiropractic, and even dentistry years ago. Such a record has disqualified it as an objective observer.

This book is not to be interpreted as an attack against the average doctor of medicine, who in general, is well meaning, dedicated and sincerely devoted to making sick people well. Of course, they have the same human frailties as the rest of us, not excepting doctors of chiropractic. To characterize physicians on the basis of the behavior of a minority of them is not fair or honest. The philosopher George Bernard Shaw summarized it well when he said, "As to the honor and conscience of doctors, they have as much as any other class of men, no more and no less."

The attitude of medical physicians toward chiropractic may vary. They may be ignorant or prejudiced from misinformation or from a lack of information. They may be indifferent. They may be favorably inclined toward chiropractic. If they are favorable to chiropractic, however, they cannot openly refer patients to a chiropractor without the possibility of being threatened by organized medicine's code of ethics which specifically denies them this right. In spite of this, a 1972 national survey of medical physicians revealed that most of them revealed that chiropractic did have a significant clinical value to patients. Only 22 per cent shared the AMA's antichiropractic position.

Medical physicians are not only exposed to the same propaganda we are, but too frequently their patients will refrain from telling them about their good results with chiropractic for fear of embarrassing or angering them. Patients will tell friends, neighbors and relatives, but family medical doctors often are the last to hear of their patients' successes with chiropractic. Here is a classic example. A nurse who worked as a medical doctor's assistant for 18 years had close contact with his patients' histories and consultations. Chiropractic was rarely mentioned to this physician by his patients. After the doctor's death the nurse started working for a doctor of chiropractic. She met many of the medical doctor's former patients. They literally swamped her with their personal testimonials about chiropractic. The former patients included some of the medical doctor's closest and dearest friends.

What a great tragedy that these people had not revealed their chiropractic experiences earlier to this physician. To withhold such information deliberately is to share the guilt of contributing to and perpetuating the ignorance and needless suffering of so many people. If patients have had help through chiropractic care, they should tell their family medical doctors in the spirit of better interprofessional understanding. How else can medical physicians learn of the benefits of chiropractic?

IS CHIROPRACTIC OR MEDICINE SCIENTIFIC?

No healing profession is exactingly scientific, and this includes medicine and chiropractic. Any profession that is could guarantee results. In fact, any physician guaranteeing results with a patient is violating his profession's code of ethics.

Patients, on admission to hospitals, often must sign release statements that they understand that the practice of medicine is not an exact science. The frequent practice of prescribing medications on the basis that it might help the patient, then having the patient return later for a different medication if the symptoms do not subside, cannot be considered entirely scientific. Furthermore, the most prescribed medication is aspirin, yet modern medicine cannot prove how it works.

One irate patient, visiting numerous medical physicians and receiving as many diagnoses and treatments, protested to the local medical society. He received the predictable answer: "We sympathize with your dilemma. Because medicine is an inexact science, it is not unusual for physicians to differ in their diagnosis of a problem, or suggestions for treatment."

The tragedy of the confusion concerning scientific health care lies in the frequent inference that chiropractic is not scientific, thereby implying that medicine *is*. Actually, both chiropractic and medicine can more accurately be described as arts, concepts and philosophies based on scientific principles.

"PINCHED NERVES"

Medical misnomers have been used by physicians in all branches of the healing arts. Though scientifically inaccurate, expressions like "pinched nerve," "slipped disc," "double joint," "thin blood," seem to provide patients an uncomplicated answer for their ailment. Instead of a "pinched nerve," could you imagine a patient being advised that they have a mechanical nerve conduction block or a proprioceptive neurovascular insult initiating nerve inhibition or facilitation? Or how would a posterior herniation of the annulus fibroses with protrusion of the nucleus pulposes into the spinal canal sound to a patient instead of a slipped disc?

These illustrations do not advocate or even defend the practice of using misnomers; it merely explains why it takes place within the healing professions.

Though "pinched nerve" is used *figuratively* by chiropractors, it is quoted *literally* by its critics. It is difficult to accept that organized medicine can be so naive as to misquote chiropractic so grossly. By literally quoting a "pinched nerve," it can provide itself with a vehicle of condemning chiropractic's premise before the scientific community. The misnomer, as used by chiropractors, and more recently by medical physicians, has provided the propagandist a tool by which he can denigrate chiropractic, and promote more ignorance and prejudice in healing.

CHIROPRACTIC'S POSITION ON DRUGS

There are great misconceptions about chiropractic's position on drugs. One frequent charge is, "Since chiropractors are not trained or permitted to prescribe medications, they try to discredit or ignore drug therapy."

The medical propagandists have deaf ears to the constant denials of this by the chiropractic profession. The propagandists nevertheless prefer to repeat these charges and, unfortunately, many persons accept them as true. Actually, chiropractors do not oppose the rational use of medications. They have imposed self restriction on the use of drugs because it is contrary to the natural principles of chiropractic. Furthermore, a physician simply cannot divide his interest into two different therapies and be as proficient in both.

In 1962, Batten and Associates conducted a national survey of chiropractors to determine if they referred patients to other doctors. The report showed that over 90 per cent of the chiropractors polled referred patients to other doctors, while 86.5 per cent referred patients to doctors of medicine. Is this the behavior of a profession which claims cure-all methods and opposes drugs?

It is always possible, of course, to find exceptions to a rule and then use these exceptions as though they constituted the rule. Such practice is common among the dishonest and unethical.

It might be noted that in a survey of medical doctors a few years ago, some five per cent felt smoking was not injurious to health. One cannot conclude from this that medicine found no link between smoking and cancer.

Along this same line there are medical doctors who claim that drugs for the cure and eradication of cancer exist, but are being withheld from the public. Based on the claims of a few licensed medical physicians would it be honest and proper to suggest or propagandize that medicine claims to have a cure for cancer? Of course not.

Chiropractors frequently have criticized the indiscriminate, abusive and excessive use of drugs and surgery by medical doctors. For this reason, some people have assumed chiropractors are generally opposed to drugs. The fact that chiropractors do not use drugs in their practice does not mean that they oppose them, in cases where the use of drugs appears necessary, they simply refer patients to doctors of medicine. Since medicine is not a cure-all either, it will be a great day for humanity when medical doctors also regularly refer patients to doctors of chiropractic.

CHIROPRACTIC AND VACCINATIONS

In 1969, organized medicine circulated a reprint which said: "Chiropractic makes strenuous efforts to raise doubts in the minds of people about the value of vaccination . . . Often, chiropractors are in the forefront of opposition to school immunization programs to prevent smallpox."

Indeed, chiropractic journals have been increasing its criticism of massive smallpox vaccination of children in recent years. Now, let's examine the facts.

Between 14 and 18 million smallpox vaccinations have been given annually in the United States. An article in the July, 1969 issue of *Prevention Magazine* states that 300 children in the United States have died from the complications of vaccination for smallpox since 1948, whereas we haven't had even a single case of smallpox reported in this country during that period. Dr. C. Henry Kemp, University of Colorado School of Medicine, said in the article: "The danger of contracting serious illness from smallpox is now greater than the danger from the disease itself. . . . Routine primary vaccination in pediatric practice can no longer be justified. . . . We haven't had a single case of smallpox in the United States in the last 20 years. In fact, if smallpox vaccine was up for licensing, at the present time, federal agencies would not sanction its manufacture and distribution because it is intended to prevent a nonexistent, nonfatal disease."

The American Academy of Pediatrics held its annual meeting in Chicago on October 23, 1971. Dr. Samuel L. Katz, chairman of the department of pediatrics, Duke University Medical Center, and chairman of the AAP's infectious committee, announced that smallpox vaccinations should no longer be given to children or adults in the United States (except for travelers to certain countries). He pointed out that an average of six to nine individuals die each year from smallpox vaccinations; in 1970, there were 12 known cases of neurological damage and 163 known instances of skin disorders resulting from smallpox vaccinations.

Thus, compulsory vaccinations should no longer be given according to the American Academy of Pediatrics, which has been joined recently in this position by the U.S. Public Health Service. State laws requiring smallpox vaccination will probably be changed or no longer enforced. Today, medicine is repeating what chiropractic has been saying all along, and for which it previously had been condemned.

The agency responsible for licensing of vaccines is the Division of Biologics Standards (DBS). It has licensed 19 vaccines; 150 million doses are given annually to the public.

Dr. J. A. Morris, a research microbiologist for the DBS, submitted a report to Senator Abraham Ribicoff on the safety and effectiveness of different vaccines. It was published October 15, 1971 in the Congressional Record. Dr. Morris' report charged that the agency released vaccines for massive public programs without sufficient testing. These included vaccines for measles, mumps, influenza and German measles.

Dr. Morris said the mumps vaccine "was certified safe by its manufacturer over the scientific doubts of some of its own researchers." Of the measles vaccine, he said the procedure for checking for cancer-causing viruses "is incapable of detecting more than a few of many known groups of such contaminating agents." He said the researcher who helped develop the first German measles vaccine refused to use it on his children because he felt another vaccine had fewer side effects. On the influenza vaccine, he said it was released for general use "before the benefits and risks associated with its use were determined." He added that the record since 1944 shows that influenza shots have not been effective in preventing the disease, and that the shots have caused harm in many people, particularly pregnant women.

Dr. Alex Shelokov, the DBS official who was responsible for assuring the safety of the influenza vaccine, stated under oath: "For many years, I have not taken influenza vaccine myself or given it to my family. I have not been impressed with its potency."

Another DBS official, Dr. Nicola Tauraso, said the drug manufacturers "would sell water if they could get away with it."

In the light of these facts, what confidence and trust can be placed in particular vaccines when their safety and effectiveness is questioned by officials and researchers of the DBS?

CHIROPRACTIC AND CANCER

Critics of chiropractic frequently quote a 1962 Batten and Associates study in which seven per cent of the chiropractors polled indicated that they treat patients with cancer. The implication is made that these chiropractors boast cancer cures. But this is not true. Chiropractors realize that the best known cure for cancer is early detection and proper medical and surgical care.

What about the terminal cancer cases who will die anyway, and find their only relief in chiropractic therapy? Should they be denied relief? Or would a joint medical-chiropractic effort be more humane? On that basis, the seven per cent figure actually is much too low. But most chiropractors are sensitive about that question; often maligned, misquoted, and quoted out of context, they simply answer that question negatively. Furthermore, since so little is known about cancer, who can say with certainty that lowered tissue resistance is not a factor in cancer?

References are made of cancer cases missed by chiropractors and later diagnosed by medical physicians. Indeed, the inverse also is true. Chiropractors can cite cases of cancer that they found in patients which were missed by medical physicians.

A study of the Boston City Hospital revealed that between 1955 and 1965 over 1,100 cases of cancer, or 26.2 per cent, went undetected by medical physicians. And there is no indication that public hospitals today would fare better under a similar study. It must be concluded in all fairness that early cancer cases often go undetected because of inadequate symptoms presented by the patients, and not necessarily due to inadequacies or errors on the part of physicians.

CHIROPRACTORS DIAGNOSE

The statement frequently has been made that "chiropractors are not trained to recognize disease or make a diagnosis."

That statement is absolutely false.

All chiropractic colleges in the United States and Canada clearly list diagnosis within their catalogues and, in fact, separate it into clinical diagnosis, laboratory diagnosis, physical diagnosis and differential diagnosis. One prominent chiropractic college surveyed showed that 43 per cent of the curriculum was devoted to differential diagnosis. The subjects of pathology and bacteriology are also a part of the standard curriculum. Before chiropractors are permitted to practice, they must pass state examinations. In the state of Illinois, for example, they must pass comprehensive three day examinations which include diagnosis, pathology, bacteriology, dermatology, neurology, anatomy, physiology, chemistry, and public health. The tests are very similar to ones given for doctors of osteopathy and medicine. Of course, doctors of medicine and osteopathy are not examined in chiropractic principles and techniques and doctors of chiropractic are not examined in surgery or pharmacology, since they do not use surgery or drugs.

The licensing of chiropractors in Illinois requires that candidates pass all subjects on which they are examined, including diagnosis. Their licenses mean that the seven-man examining board has concluded that they have demonstrated reasonable proficiency to be licensed to practice chiropractic, which includes diagnosing illnesses as well as spinal examinations. To say otherwise is a direct insult to this medical board of examiners which is composed of five medical doctors, one doctor of osteopathy, and one doctor of chiropractic. Furthermore, it is an insult to the examining boards in 50 states, the District of Columbia and Puerto Rico.

U.S. OFFICE OF EDUCATION

Statements have been circulated that the degree of doctor of chiropractic is designated as "spurious" by the U.S. Office of Education. Webster's dictionary defines spurious as, illegitimate, false, bastardly and counterfeit. This certainly would be a serious condemnation of the doctor of chiropractic degree by the U.S. Office of Education, had it actually labeled the degree "spurious." Here is what really happened and how propagandists were able to make that charge.

The U.S. Office of Education publication entitled, *Academic Degrees* listed the chiropractic degree as "spurious" and "valid" within the same publication in an obvious error. On page 236 of that publication it was listed as "spurious," but on page 169 of the same publication it was listed as "valid." Obviously it could not be both. It would be the same as a woman saying she was a "wee bit pregnant." She either is or she isn't; she can't be both.

The senior author of that publication, Dr. Walter Crosby Eells, wrote to the chiropractic profession on January 16, 1961, that the listing of the D.C. degree as spurious was an unfortunate error. In the letter he specifically stated: "The printing of it in Roman type on page 169 (as a valid degree) is the correct one."

In 1969 the National Council of Senior Citizens published in its January issue of its newspaper the erroneous statement. Organized medicine promptly circulated reprints of this statement to key members of Congress in an effort to denigrate chiropractic. Although organized medicine collaborated with the *Senior Citizen News* in writing the article, it propagandized to the congressmen that the article came from an independent nonmedical source. The exact wording of the half-truth within a bold, boxed-off section said: "Did You Know? Doctors of Chiropractic degrees (D.C.) are listed as 'spurious' by the U.S. Office of Education in a recent publication entitled *Academic Degrees.*" This statement, if not a deliberate misrepresentation, indicates that organized medicine is inadequate in researching the facts objectively and correctly.

EDUCATIONAL REQUIREMENTS OF CHIROPRACTORS

A frequent misconception about chiropractic, which has been spread by propagandists, is that anyone can go to a chiropractic college 18 months and become a chiropractor.

This is simply not true. Not one chiropractic college in the United States or Canada accepts applicants without at least a high school diploma and two years of college credits. None of the chiropractic colleges in existence has less than a four-year curricula. A four-year chiropractic course averages 4,485 hours which compares with medical schools.

Most states require at least two years of extra professional college plus four years professional college for license application. The state legislatures which have enacted higher educational requirements for chiropractic were supported by the chiropractic profession within that state. This type of action documents the profession's drive for highest possible educational standards.

The educational requirements for state licensure of chiropractic, as of 1976, are given below. These requirements are a matter of state public record. Chiropractors cannot practice in these states unless they meet these requirements and pass state examinations.

THE DIPLOMA MILLS

In August of 1923, reporter Harry Thompson Brundige of the *St. Louis Star,* was assigned to do an exposé on medical diploma mills. The newspaper had reason to believe that the then defunct National University of Arts and Sciences in St. Louis, was for some time selling medical degrees, and that

UNITED STATES

Jurisdiction	*Nonprofessional Education Required*	*Profesional Education Required*	*Type of Examining Board*
Alabama	High School	4 yrs. of 9 mo. each	†C
Alaska	H. S. & 2 yrs. College	4 yrs. of 9 mo. each	†C
Arizona	High School	4 yrs. of 9 mo. each	†C
Arkansas	H. S. & 2 yrs. College	4 yrs. of 9 mo. each	†C-B
California	High School	4 yrs. of 9 mo. each	C
Colorado	High School	4 yrs.—4,000 hours	†C-B
Connecticut	H. S. & 2 yrs. College	4 yrs. of 8 mo. each—4,000 hours	C
Delaware	H. S. & 2 yrs. College	4 yrs. of 8 mo. each	†C
Dist. of Columbia	H. S. & 2 yrs. College	4 yrs. of 9 mo. each	†C-B
Florida	H. S. & 2 yrs. College	4 yrs.—4,000 hours	†C
Georgia	H. S. & 2 yrs. College	4 yrs. of 9 mo. each	C
Hawaii	H. S. & 2 yrs. College	4 yrs. of 9 mo. each	†C
Idaho	H. S. & 2 yrs. College	4 yrs. of 8 mo. each	†C
Illinois	H. S. & 2 yrs. College	4 yrs. of 8 mo. each	MX
Indiana	H. S. & 2 yrs. College	4 yrs.—4,000 hours	MX
Iowa	High School	4 yrs.—4,000 hours	†C
Kansas	H. S. & 2 yrs. College	4 yrs. of 9 mo. each	†MX
Kentucky	H. S. & 2 yrs. College	4 yrs. of 9 mo. each—4,000 hours	†C
Louisiana	H. S. & 2 yrs. College	4 yrs. of 9 mo. each	†C
Maine	H. S. & 2 yrs. College	4 yrs.—4,400 hours	†C
Maryland	H. S. & 2 yrs. College	4 yrs.—4,000 hours	C

UNITED STATES (*Continued*)

Jurisdiction	*Nonprofessional Education Required*	*Professional Education Required*	*Type of Examining Board*
Massachusetts	H. S. & 2 yrs. College	4 yrs.—4,000 hours	†MX
Michigan	H. S. & 2 yrs. College	4 yrs. of 9 mo. each	†C
Minnesota	H. S. & 2 yrs. College	4 yrs. of 8 mo. each—4,000 hours	†C
Mississippi	H. S.	4 yrs. of 9 mo. each	†MX
Missouri	H. S.	3 yrs. of 9 mo. each	†C
Montana	H. S. & 2 yrs. College	4 yrs. of 9 mo. each	†C
Nebraska	H. S. & 2 yrs. College	4 yrs.—4,000 hours	†C
Nevada	H. S. & 2 yrs. College	4 yrs.—4,000 hours	†C
New Hampshire	High School	4 yrs.—3,600 hours	†C
New Jersey	H. S. & 2 yrs. College	4 yrs. of 9 mo. each	†MX
New Mexico	H. S. & 2 yrs. College	4 yrs. of 4,000 hours	†C
New York	H. S. & 2 yrs. College	4 yrs. of 8 mo. each—4,000 hrs.	†MX
North Carolina	H. S. & 2 yrs. College	4 yrs. of 9 mo. each	†C
North Dakota	H. S. & 2 yrs. College	4 yrs. of 8 mo. each	†C
Ohio	H. S. & 2 yrs. College	4 yrs. of 9 mo. each—4,000 hrs.	C
Oklahoma	H. S. & 2 yrs. College	4 yrs. of 9 mo. each—4,150 hrs.	C
Oregon	H. S. & 2 yrs. College	4 yrs. of 9 mo. each	†C
Pennsylvania	H. S. & 1 yr. College	4 yrs. of 9 mo. each	†C
Puerto Rico	H. S. & 2 yrs. College	4 yrs. of 9 mo. each	C
Rhode Island	H. S. & 2 yrs. College	4 yrs. of 8 mo. each	†C
South Carolina	High School	4 yrs. of 9 mo. each	†C
South Dakota	H. S. & 2 yrs. College	4 yrs. of 9 mo. each	†C

Tennessee	H. S. & 2 yrs. College	4 yrs. of 9 mo. each	C
Texas	H. S. & 2 yrs. College	4 yrs. of 8 mo. each	C-B
Utah	H. S. & 1 yr. College	4 yrs. of 8½ mo. each—4,000 hrs.	†C-B
Vermont	H. S. & 2 yrs. College	4 yrs.—3,600 hrs.	†C
Virginia	H. S. & 2 yrs. College	4 yrs. of 8 mo. each	†MX
Washington	High School	4,000 hours	†C-B
West Virginia	H. S. & 2 yrs. College	4 yrs. of 9 mo. each—4,000 hours	†C
Wisconsin	H. S. & 2 yrs. College	4 yrs. of 9 mo. each	†C
Wyoming	H. S. & 2 yrs. College	4 yrs. of 9 mo. each	†C
CANADA			
Alberta	Junior Matriculation	4 yrs. of 8 mo. each	*C
British Columbia	1 yr. College	4 yrs. of 8 mo. each & 1 yr. University	*C
Manitoba	Junior Matriculation	4 academic years	*C
New Brunswick	Senior Matriculation	4 yrs. of 9 mo. each	*C
Ontario	Grade XIII	4 yrs. of 9 mo. each—4,200 hrs.	*C
Prince Edward Island	Not specified	Approved college	*C
Saskatchewan	Senior Matriculation	4 yrs. of 8 mo. each	*C
Nova Scotia	Senior Matriculation	4 yrs. of 8 mo. each	*C
Quebec	D. E. C. Health Option		*C
Yukon Territory	Must hold license from either province or Oregon or Washington		*C

Symbols designating Boards: C—Chiropractic. C-B—Chiropractic & Basic Science. MD—Medical. MX—Mixed (Composed of medical and chiropractic members).

† Recognize or utilize National Board of Chiropractic Examiners Certificate. (Some additional states consider on an individual basis).

* Recognize examinations of Canadian Chiropractic Examining Board.

numerous physicians in St. Louis and Kansas City were involved.

Posing as a coal salesman by the name of Harry Thompson, the reporter rented a room two doors west of Dr. Robert Adcox, a prominent physician suspected of being involved in the diploma mill racket. Making friends with the doctor, the reporter was told that he could obtain a medical diploma for about $1,000.

They left for Kansas City, where they met Dr. Ralph A. Voight, who assured Thompson of a high school certificate, a medical diploma and a state license. Voight suggested that Thompson start with the senior year at the Kansas City College of Medicine and Surgery, in order to have a cursory knowledge of medicine. Thompson rejected the idea saying that his total ignorance of medicine would be easily recognized in a senior class. But Voight assured him that the professors would not ask any questions. He said, "You'll be in a ringer class. The professor will put you on the list with the others who are there to listen and not to answer questions."

Thompson insisted on not going to school, and on October 3, 1923, Voight gave the diploma to Thompson, along with a license to practice in the state of Tennessee. However, erasure marks on the license made it unacceptable to Thompson, and Voight agreed to provide other documents.

While waiting for his medical diploma and state license, Thompson also went ahead with his plans to obtain a chiropractic diploma. With the assistance of Dr. Voight, he received his diploma from the Progressive College of Chiropractic in Chicago, Illinois. It came by way of Dr. D. R. Alexander, Dean of the Kansas City College of Medicine and Surgery. Dr. Henry Lindlahr, the founder and president of the chiropractic college, was not even a chiropractor. He was a graduate of the National Medical University.

Finally, Thompson's medical degree arrived from the Department of Medicine, National University of Arts and Sciences, St. Louis, Missouri. Also, he received a high school certificate signed by the state superintendent of public instruction in Missouri. His certificate and diploma were predated to a time before the National University had closed its doors.

On October 15, 1923, the *St. Louis Star* broke the story in a series of articles. One of the articles revealed how Voight, confiding in Thompson, said his most difficult job was to "take 42 boobs to New Haven (Conn.) to get licenses for them." He paid $1,500 for an advance copy of the examination questions, then stayed up all night with his applicants writing answers. Voight said, "We prepared 42 different sets of answers, one for each boob, and all they had to do was go into the examination room and copy the answers in their own handwriting. Only one failed to get his license—a dumb bird who could not copy his paper!"

The exposé resulted in 167 physicians having their licenses revoked in Connecticut. Drs. Voight, Adcox and Alexander were all arrested. Professor Sachs, former examiner of the Missouri schools also was arrested. Sachs confessed, "I sold approximately 5,000 of these certificates, directly or indirectly, to persons who could not have passed the examinations but later became doctors of medicine."

Indeed, medical and chiropractic diploma mills have existed years ago. Unfortunately, medical propagandists have dwelled on the ones in chiropractic, while conspicuously avoiding references to those in medicine. The last and most recent attempt to open a fly-by-night chiropractic college in America was stopped through the efforts of the chiropractic profession. No group of persons are more strenuously opposed to the opening of such a diploma mill than chiropractors, because it would prostitute the standards of a profession striving for excellence and greater recognition.

Organized medicine heavily promotes an antichiropractic propaganda mass market paperback book which, among other false charges, makes the statement, "In 1945 *Medical World News* reported that it was still possible to obtain a mail order doctor of chiropractic degree from a Chicago college for

$127.50." The AMA's Department of Investigation sent copies of the book to state and county medical societies, and hardbound copies to the 1,200 largest libraries in the nation. It urged physicians to purchase large quantities of the book for distribution to their patients.

Actually, it was impossible for *Medical World News* to make any kind of a statement in 1945 since it did not exist at that time. It was first published in 1960. Furthermore, *Medical World News* found no record of ever making reference to a chiropractic mail order diploma.

Chiropractic education today requires many years of training before an applicant qualifies to take a state examination for licensure. Even in the 1940s, state licensing bodies would not accept such diplomas. However, the real tragedy of such a statement is that uninformed persons believe what they read and are discouraged from seeking the services of chiropractors with the belief that the chiropractor's education is inadequate.

RAN ITS COURSE

The critics of chiropractic, in an effort to explain its great success with patients, have said: "Many conditions are self limiting; in other words, patients would have improved anyway, while chiropractors were credited with getting the results."

Many chronic sufferers who did not respond to extensive medical treatment have found quick, effective and dramatic results under chiropractic care. Some of these patients were suffering 10 or 20 years or longer. Common sense indicates that all these chronic and long standing cases could not suddenly "run their course" following chiropractic care. Too many such cases are documented.

Why did the Florida Industrial Commission survey show that the average patient under chiropractic care returned to work in three days compared to nine days under medical care? Assuming the chiropractic patients all "ran their course" in three days, why did the medical patients with similar neck and back conditions take nine days? Are we to assume on that basis that the medical care prolonged the average illness by six more days? Statistically, the patients returned to work three times sooner under chiropractic care than under medical care for the same type of conditions.

Other state as well as national workmen's compensation surveys provide supportive evidence of this finding. These documented facts not only refute the "run its course" theory but help to validate the effectiveness of chiropractic.

People have been diagnosed by medical physicians as needing surgery of the spine, only to turn to chiropractic care and experience complete recovery. Adequate clinical documentation supports this fact. Television star John Gary is one of many examples (see chapter 18).

Finally, chiropractic has built its reputation on medical failures, on people who could not be helped through medical means.

IT'S ALL IN YOUR MIND

In searching for excuses for the great success of chiropractic, another argument offered is: Patients who were helped through chiropractic received psychosomatic suggestions; in other words, it was all in their minds.

Could you imagine telling some rugged truck driver, bricklayer, or other laborer that the sudden pain and muscle spasm he felt in his back as he was bending and lifting, and which was corrected after visiting a chiropractor, was "all in his mind?"

Very often the patient has had psychosomatic suggestions by several medical physicians before going to a chiropractor. Finally, as a last resort the patient approached the chiropractor with reluctance, skepticism, defiance, practically challenging him to prove himself worthy of the patient's confidence—AND THE CHIROPRACTOR GOT RESULTS.

This was certainly not the climate for psychosomatic suggestion.

Dr. Neville Ussher, a medical researcher at the Santa Barbara Clinic, corrected hundreds of visceral conditions in patients without drugs and through spinal manipulation only. He purposely avoided mentioning to his patients why he was manipulating the spine because he wanted to eliminate any possible psychosomatic suggestion.

Many chiropractic patients experience a general improvement in their health, this in addition to the improvement for the specific conditions for which they were treated. Since they were not even expecting other health improvements, no psychosomatic influences would be likely.

Finally, clinical results with children under chiropractic care who were too young to be influenced by psychosomatic suggestion, further disprove the argument.

CHIROPRACTIC PROVEN SAFE

Some people have shown a reluctance in consulting a chiropractor because of a fear based on erroneous information disseminated by propagandists. Based on malpractice insurance rates, however, chiropractic is a far safer insurance risk than medicine. As of September, 1971, the United States Fidelity and Guaranty Company using the Insurance Services Office figures, revealed the following standard annual premium rates for $100,000/$300,000 liability limits for orthopedists. In Chicago it was $2,022, New York was $5,477, and in Los Angeles it was $5,783. And the trend is worsening. The 1972 Insurance Services Office figures for the same insurance coverage in New York increased to $6,773, in Los Angeles it increased to $6,369. The 1976 I.S.O. figures for the same insurance coverage in New York increased to $25,134, and in Los Angeles increased to $49,417.63.

The Wall Street Journal, January 6, 1971, reported medical doctors were having difficulty getting their malpractice insurance renewed because the insurance companies were losing money by insuring them, even at such high premium rates. President Nixon told Congress in 1971 that a "climate of fear" is surrounding medical physicians because of the "growing menace of malpractice suits."

Meanwhile chiropractic insurance rates are about 1/50th of the above costs for medicine, making chiropractic's rates modest by comparison, to say the least.

The insurance companies make it their business to know the liability risk of the insured. Their existence depends on the accuracy of actuarial reports, which are devoid of sentimentality. These companies rely on cold hard facts, figures and statistics, and objective conclusions. What greater proof of the safe method of chiropractic therapy can be demonstrated than the low malpractice premium rates of doctors of chiropractic as compared to higher malpractice premium rates of doctors of medicine? Insurance rates speaks for themselves!

The next time a medical critic makes a statement that chiropractic represents a significant health hazard, ask him why chiropractic malpractice rates are 50 times less expensive than for comparable medical coverage. These documented insurance rates reduce such statements to the point of being ludicrous.

CHIROPRACTIC AND MEDICAL MALPRACTICE

Malpractice suits against chiropractors, as compared to medical physicians, are relatively rare. Yet, critics seem to dwell on the exceptional cases in chiropractic. Some of the most vicious attacks against chiropractic have been based on the case of a young California girl who died of cancer of the eye while being treated by a chiropractor in 1961. The suggestion is that chiropractic is plagued with many similar cases. Even though the guilt of some of the doctors is questionable, nevertheless it makes for sensational reading and attempts to demean the entire chiropractic profession.

Since the antagonists of chiropractic choose to cite a California case against chiropractic, let's use the same state in another study. Dr. George H. Haynes, from the Los Angeles College of Chiropractic, found that during a six month period ending May 20, 1970, 35 alleged law violations by doctors of medicine occurred in California. These included fraud, narcotics violation, illegal abortions, forgery, morals, rape, assault and battery, murder, income tax evasions, and false claims of cures.

Medical malpractice suits during the same period in California, concerned death due to negligence, negligence during delivery, permanent injury following therapeutic abortion, radiation burns, errors during surgery (wrong area or objects left in patient), injury due to medication, improper vasectomy, and permanent injury due to surgery or improper treatment. The suits asked damages of more than $47 million. The amount paid out in claims during that period was $1,680,010.

Eli Burnsweig, director of the United States Department of Health, Education, and Welfare's Advisory Commission on Medical Malpractice, said there are probably over 10,000 malpractice suits a year against medical doctors, with the figure increasing at the rate of 10 per cent a year. Claims against medical physicians have been rising so rapidly during the past five years, President Nixon has ordered that a commission on malpractice be formed to examine the problem.

On December 17, 1971, Dr. Sidney Wolfe, a representative of Ralph Nader's research group, testified before the commission on medical malpractice. He said that at least 10,000 Americans die as a result of the two million unnecessary surgical operations each year. These include 250 deaths from unnecessary tonsillectomies and adenoidectomies, 500 deaths from unnecessary appendectomies, and another 500 deaths from unnecessary hysterectomies. Dr. Wolfe said further that the rising number of malpractice suits "offers partial testimony to the incompetence of doctors as to proper diagnosis and treatment of disease."

Charles Kramer, prominent attorney and author of *The Negligent Doctor*, said there is ten times more malpractice committed by medical physicians than there are malpractice cases.

It is estimated by Senator Abraham Ribicoff that nearly one out of five of all U.S. medical physicians have been defendants in malpractice suits, and in some metropolitan areas the ratio is estimated at one out of three. Statistics show that average settlements exceed $13,000.

Senator Abraham Ribicoff's Subcommittee on Executive Reorganization in 1969 reported: Most malpractice suits are the direct result of injuries suffered by patients during medical treatment or surgery. The majority have proved justifiable." The report also added, "The situation now threatens to become a national crisis."

An executive secretary of a state medical association said, "In discipline, we ought to be called disorganized medicine." Most state medical societies have adopted weak disciplinary provisions, rarely consulting one another, while the AMA is not prepared to act as a clearing house.

A study conducted by Dr. R. C. Derbyshire of the Federation of State Medical Boards, revealed that only eight state medical societies can take action against a mentally or professionally incompetent member. During the five years preceding the study, only seven charges of incompetence were reported.

Daniel Hoffman, a Denver attorney specializing in medical malpractice cases, addressed the Colorado Medical Society and said: "Total lack of adequate internal policing is partly to blame for the soaring number of malpractice suits against the medics. Physicians who are alcoholics, drug addicts, mentally unstable, or medically incompetent are allowed to practice in Colorado because the state's medical profession has failed to discipline itself. . . . Never once has a Colorado doctor had his license revoked for medical incompetence—in fact, I know of only three such cases in the entire country."

The fact that malpractice insurance premiums for physicians and surgeons can be more than 50 times higher than for chiropractors illustrates the low incidence of malpractice within chiropractic.

Many dramatic stories could be told of medical negligence and incompetence. They could be melodramatically presented in this book with all the gory details. To do so, however, would make us guilty of the same dishonest tactics as are the antagonists of the chiropractic profession.

LACK OF REFERRAL—A POTENTIAL DANGER

Critics of chiropractic often have repeated a similar statement: "Chiropractic can be potentially dangerous by delaying proper medical treatment." Actually, any profession can be potentially dangerous by delaying proper treatment. Indeed, medicine can be potentially dangerous by denying proper chiropractic care.

Compression subluxations of peripheral nerves, such as sciatic nerve root compressions, can cause permanent irreversible damage if not treated in time. Dr. Bourdillon, an internationally prominent British orthopedic surgeon, noted that trophic changes can occur in a wrist or hand if a patient is delayed proper neck and upper back spinal manipulation. He added that in 15 years in a busy practice he did not see any secondary trophic changes except among patients medically treated elsewhere, where the syndrome was allowed to develop before the neck was properly treated. Once the changes in the distal part became advanced, he noted, they were not easily reversed.

Annually, nearly 1½ million people are hospitalized, and 100,000 die as a result of medication reaction. How many of these cases could have been avoided by referrals to chiropractors? How many unnecessary disc operations, which resulted in permanent injury or death, could have been prevented?

Using the figures of Dr. Virgil Slee of the Commission on Professional and Hospital Activities, there were 20,000,000 operations performed in 1971. Conservative estimates indicate that one out of five operations have been unnecessary. This would imply 4,000,000 unnecessary operations. Using the major surgery mortality rate of 1.2 per cent, an estimated 48,000 persons died from needless surgery in 1971.

Critics can sight isolated chiropractic cases in which proper medical attention was denied. But what about the medical cases above? This does not imply that chiropractic would have had all the answers. But it certainly does stress the need for an objective and unbiased cooperation between these two professions. Unfortunately, the cooperation seems to be more unilateral, with chiropractors doing most of the referring. Therefore, if an assessment is to be made concerning the lack of proper interprofessional patient referral with resultant patient injury, the blame must fall principally upon the shoulders of orthodox medicine.

THE TARDINESS OF LOUISIANA

The practice of chiropractic was not licensed or regulated in Louisiana until June, 1974. Thus, any person with a chiropractic diploma could have opened an office there without passing a qualifying examination. It also meant that Louisiana did not specify any educational requirements for a person with a chiropractic diploma. Therefore, it encouraged the opening of a totally unapproved "fly-by-night" chiropractic college. The danger of such a college getting started was a genuine one. A charter could have been acquired under state sanction to teach a totally inadequate and inferior course of studies. To prevent such colleges from opening, Louisiana had to adopt laws for the licensing and regulation of chiropractic. In doing so the state could set adequate educational requirements for a chiropractor.

The unlicensing situation existed until 1974, but not because the chiropractic profession wanted it. Louisiana and Mississippi chiropractors repeatedly attempted to get legislation providing for strict licensing and regulation of chiropractic in these states, and Mississippi "won" by offering a licensing program in 1973. Strong medical opposition had been exerted by organized medicine because it would rather see chiropractic as a back door operation than permit it to have the respectability of state recognition, high standards and patient protection.

Ironically, if such a diploma mill had ever opened its doors, organized medicine in its customary and bigoted display of concern for the public welfare, would have been first to bring it into public attention in demeaning of the entire chiropractic profession. Most of the earlier propaganda articles seldom missed an opportunity to mention that chiropractic was not licensed and regulated in Louisiana and Mississippi.

As you would drive along highways in Louisiana, you could encounter billboards which read: "THE SHAME OF LOUISIANA." The smaller print would tell you that it was sponsored by the chiropractic profession in Louisiana. In its desperate effort to obtain legislation and assure the highest possible standards of chiropractic, it had taken the issue to the court of last resort, the people.

After numerous and futile attempts to license and regulate chiropractic through the Louisiana legislature, the chiropractic profession took the issue to the courts. It was unsuccessful after a long and bitter struggle.

Much antichiropractic literature refers to *England v. Louisiana State Board of Medical Examiners*, 5th Cir., 259F. 2d 626 (1958). And generally such statistics quote only a part of the U.S. District Court decision that it wants the reader to see. For example, a statement of the AMA House of Delegates contained the following paragraph:

> "In 1965, a United States District Court, in upholding a state's right (constitutional) to refuse to license chiropractors, said that 'since chiropractic claims to be a complete and independent healing art capable of curing almost all kinds of disease, the state Legislature may have felt that a requirement of a foundation in materia medica and surgery. . . . would be a protection to the public.' "

Immediately following the above quote, the AMA delegate statement added, "Without dissent, the United States Supreme Court affirmed the decision." Also, the September 15, 1969, Journal of the AMA repeated that "the earlier decision by a three-judge federal court that was affirmed by the U.S. Supreme Court . . ."

It is a fact that the U.S. Supreme Court did not affirm the decision of the district court. The Supreme Court did not even hear the case. The U.S. Supreme Court refused to hear the case and therefore did not comment on it. Thus, even the medical physician reading his own journal is not getting the true story.

The U.S. District Court held that the State of Louisiana had a right to establish its own standards for professional people. It was purely a question of constitutionality (states' rights), and cannot be interpreted as supporting or rejecting the Louisiana Supreme Court decision.

Conspicuously excluded from the AMA statement is a part

of that same United States District Court decision which says: "It may well be that chiropractic is a useful profession and that the requirement of a medical education is not in the public interest. But the balancing of the advantages and disadvantages of this requirement is for the legislature."

In summary, chiropractors in Louisiana insisted that since they do not use drugs or surgery in their therapy, a course in materia medica and surgery and a medical degree for licensing was not necessary or of concern to the public. The federal court ruled that this issue was not within its jurisdiction, and that it was for the state court to decide. The U.S. Supreme Court by not hearing an appeal did, in effect, support the district court. From these facts medical propagandists skillfully created classic examples of half-truths.

Fortunately, public and legislative support mounted for the licensing of chiropractic in Louisiana to such an extent, that the licensing of chiropratic finally took place in June, 1974.

THE WISCONSIN TASK FORCE REPORT

In 1972, a 40 man governor's task force was appointed to evaluate the health care system in Wisconsin. It consisted of numerous committees which studied specific areas of health care. The committees reported their findings and recommendations to the task force which, after approving the committee reports, made recommendations to the governor.

The expressed purpose of the task force was to help create a better understanding of the state's health needs and be able to recommend necessary health legislation. Also, the task force stated that it could help create a better understanding of chiropractic.

The chiropractic profession had mixed emotions about the study. Some chiropractors, remembering the nefarious HEW report, were apprehensive. Others felt that the task force displayed a genuine and unbiased desire for better interprofessional understanding. Thus, the Wisconsin Chiropractic Association agreed to participate in the study.

The study, "Report of the Chiropractic Study Committee to the Governor's Health Planning and Policy Task Force," was released October 23, 1972. It charged that chiropractic had no scientific validity and was a potential hazard. It recommended that chiropractic be excluded from any and all health insurance (including workmen's compensation) and from the use of public resources.

Dr. David J. Carlson, president of the Medical Society of Milwaukee County, commented on the task force report: "The demonstrated integrity of the task force and its committee assigned to investigate chiropractic is applauded by the medical profession. . . . The task force study and conclusion are ever more noteworthy in light of the fact that they represent an unbiased opinion of the task force which cannot be accused of self-interest."

The preceding information is perhaps the way the story will be told in medical journals and among biased or uninformed publications. Now, let's add some significant and documented facts, the type which are conspicuously omitted above.

The "unbiased" 40 man task force included the executive secretary of the Wisconsin State Medical Society, an attorney who is the brother of the president of the state medical society, 11 medical doctors (not one chiropractor was permitted to participate), a builder of medical clinics, representatives of the medically controlled Blue Cross-Blue Shield, two hospital administrators, one pharmacist, three medical nurses and a member of the dental society. Obviously, it was about as unbiased as a Genghis Khan Council meeting.

The three-man committee selected to study and evaluate chiropractic included a professor of pharmacology. Of course, the close tie between medicine and pharmacology is indisputable, since neither can survive without the other. The committee's evaluation of chiropractic education was based on a cursory examination of only one of eight chiropractic colleges recognized in Wisconsin. In fact, the committee actually bypassed one chiropractic college on its journey to the more distant school.

The task force report repeatedly quoted statements from a biased HEW report on chiropractic, which already had been previously rejected by Congress. Yet, it made no reference to chiropractic's "White Paper" which refuted these statements. No reference was made of the educational requirements for accreditation as established by the Association of Chiropractic Colleges or Council on Chiropractic Education. In fact, Dr. Orville Hidde, president of the Council on Chiropractic Education (coincidentally, a Wisconsin resident) made numerous attempts to contribute information to the task force. It was ignored and rejected. No pro-chiropractic statistical studies of various state workmen's compensation records, such as Florida, Colorado, Iowa and Minnesota were used. No reference was made of a two-year California old age security program showing favorable results with 39,253 chiropractic patients. No reference was made to the pro-chiropractic testimonies of 19 insurance companies which wrote 44 per cent of all the commercial health insurance premiums in the United States.

In short, the task force report conspicuously avoided complimentary information on chiropractic, except that the chiropractors were "gracious, sincere, dedicated and cooperative." Such compliments could have been submitted to serve as disclaimers of any bias, malice or contempt toward chiropractic.

The task force report acknowledged that of the nearly 5,000 questionnaires submitted to the MDs, osteopaths and chiropractors, only 1500 were "usable responses." Incredibly, the report confessed, "the number of actual responses was much higher, but we must regretfully acknowledge that a substantial number were lost in an apparently unavoidable accident." The report estimated a loss of "between 1000 and 1500" questionnaires.

The Wisconsin State Medical Society, one of the six remaining state medical societies which has not yet severed its direct ties with the AMA, appears to be serving its mother organization for propaganda purposes. The report, supported by the Wisconsin State Medical Society, is a mockery of the procedures in academic and scientific evaluation, and appears to be a last desperate propaganda attempt of organized medicine's losing battle with chiropractic.

The Wisconsin State Medical Society made a public announcement that it was assessing each of its members $10 to raise a war chest to combat chiropractic. Pressure tactics were used to extract money from the practicing medical physicians. Physicians refusing to support this endeavor received the following letter from the state society's president:

> Dear Doctor:
> This is our fourth and final request of you to pay the $10 special assessment unanimously approved by the House of Delegates last May.
> Failure to pay it means loss of your membership in your county, state and national medical societies, loss of your right to participate in the society's group health insurance plan and the group disability coverage, and the many other benefits of your society to you, your patients and your profession. You should also know that some professional liability carriers may require society membership as a condition for continuation of your protection.
> Your decision is a serious one, and I send you this letter by certified mail to be certain your decision is an informed one.

The same letter revealed an apparent "sweetheart" relationship between the Wisconsin State Medical Society and the Governor's Health Planning and Policy Task Force when it added, "Let me tell you just one aspect you may not know about this matter of educating the public on chiropractic. As your president and along with other officers, I met with Health Task Force chairman Dave Carley, and Attorney Gilda Shellow about many very important issues affecting health and medicine. We talked at length about chiropractic. Our special committee on this subject held meetings with Mrs. Shellow and her task force committee on chiropractic. We carefully gathered and presented voluminous documentation of our beliefs. Now I want you to read the enclosed report these nonmedical people presented to the task force. And they won unanimous adoption of its recommendations! It will only take a few minutes of your time, but I think you will agree that it is a remarkable and powerful document—due at least in part to the efforts of your society."

The March 28, 1973 *Milwaukee Journal* announced that the governor had addressed the state legislature concerning his health task force recommendations. He was apparently uninfluenced by the maneuvers of the Wisconsin State Medical Society, since he conspicuously excluded from his recommendations any reference to the chiropractic portion of the report.

CHAPTER V

The Tools of the Propagandists

"Sin has many tools, but a lie is the handle that fits them all."
OLIVER WENDELL HOLMES, M.D.

THE overall image of chiropractic, as created by organized medicine, can be summarized by the infamous words of Adolf Hitler: "The size of the lie is a definite factor in causing it to be believed, for the vast masses of a nation are in the depths of their hearts more easily deceived than they are consciously and intentionally bad. The primitive simplicity of their minds renders them a more easy prey to a big lie than a small one, for they themselves often tell little lies but would be ashamed to tell big ones."

When a writer conspicuously avoids the good that can be said about a subject and dwells at length on the bad, his material must be viewed with suspicion and distrust. When an author abandons objectivity, relies upon half-truths, innuendoes, exceptions to the rule, obscure sources, obsolete material, material out of context and fallacious material in an effort to derogate his subject, honesty and decency are outraged and the reader's intelligence is insulted as a lie replaces the truth. This chapter will discuss some of these tools, and how they are used by propagandists.

INNUENDOES

An innuendo is a statement that may imply something derogatory. It may hint at or insinuate something without actually coming right out and saying it. Literature castigating chiropractic has made the statement: "If you are sick go to a physician who is licensed by the state board of medical examiners." The reader's natural reaction is that chiropractors are not licensed or recognized by law, which is exactly what the propagandist wants you to believe.

Another favorite innuendo of the medical propagandist is that "chiropractors operate in the various states." Actually, chiropractors "practice" throughout the nation while the term "operate" implies something shady, dubious and deceiving. The truth is, and it can be documented by checking with your state department of registration, that chiropractors are licensed and recognized by state laws to practice in the same manner as doctors of medicine, optometry, podiatry, osteopathy or dentistry.

The January 24, 1972 *American Medical News* carried the statement: "According to the latest count, 40 states have some provisions for payment of chiropractic services under workmen's compensation."

The innuendo was that chiropractic services were rejected by workmen's compensation in 10 states. But this was not true.

Back in 1972, chiropractic services were provided by statute in 30 states, by administrative ruling of board of commission in 10 states, by court decision in one state, and at the discretion of insurance companies in the other states.

The same *American Medical News* article also carried the statement, "At least two states, New Mexico and Connecticut, have discontinued payments for chiropractic services under Medicaid." The text in which that statement was made implied that improprieties or inadequacies of chiropractors, resulted in their loss of Medicaid in some states. Again, this was simply not true. Connecticut had considered economic cutbacks in its Medicaid program, but decided to retain its same coverage, including chiropractic. New Mexico, on the other hand, did eliminate certain medical care, which included nursing homes, podiatric and chiropractic coverage. It did so as an economic cut-back which had no reflection upon any of these medical services. Thus, innocent or obsolete information taken out of context, provided the propagandist with his innuendoes.

EXCEPTIONS TO THE RULE

It is not difficult to find cases of incompetence, indiscretion or unethical practices within any healing profession. It is also not difficult to find some relatively unknown doctors whose ideas are radically different from those of their colleagues. To quote these exceptions and to imply it is typical of an entire profession is certainly dishonest and unfair. Yet, this method is widely used by propagandists.

OBSOLETE MATERIAL

The propagandist can mislead people by referring to a statement from some obsolete source of information. For example, one propaganda publication supported by organized medicine said: "Twenty-two states now require chiropractic to have one or two years college credits in addition to its chiropractic education." This is a misleading statement. It would have been more accurate if the publication replaced "twenty-two states" with thirty-seven states. Even then it wouldn't be fair to say "one or two years" preprofessional college credits because of the predominance of the two year requirement. In 1972, thirty-five states required two years extraprofessional college, while only two require one year. However, regardless of outdated or obsolete state laws, all chiropractic colleges require a minimum of two years of preprofessional college for entrance.

The propagandist may quote an absolete statement made by a chiropractor and imply it is the current or recent thinking of the chiropractic profession. We could quote many old medical errors which ridiculed and rejected sanitary procedures in obstetrics, antiseptic and sterile procedures in surgery, and sunshine and fresh air as essential for the treatment of tuberculosis. Wouldn't it be ludicrous to present these as representing the modern thinking of medicine today? It certainly would. Yet, as incredible as it may seem, this is precisely what many propagandists have done so frequently with chiropractic.

MATERIAL OUT OF CONTEXT AND HALF-TRUTHS

It is an old propaganda trick to remove a selected statement from a written or oral presentation and, without giving the entire information surrounding that statement, create a completely different meaning or attitude toward that statement. For example, someone may present a seminar on office and patient management to a group of chiropractors. Within this seminar he may stress the necessity of "being in love" with all his patients as well as with humanity. The propagandist, supported by organized medicine, can then quote out of context certain aspects of such a seminar, comparing it with "hippie love." But this is not in the usual sense of the love that a person may have for his wife or sweetheart, but rather in the spirit of compassion and total dedication to his patients and to humanity. The person presenting the seminar may stress that all these feelings must be genuine otherwise they cannot ring true and the patient will sense the falseness. It is the kind of love Hippocrates, the father of medicine, meant when he said, "For when there is the love of man, there is also love of the art."

The person presenting the seminar may also mention some public relations methods to offset the adverse literature used against chiropractic, which is common knowledge to most of us. The propagandists will falsely interpret that to mean that chiropractors are more salesmen than doctors. Common sense dictates that salesmanship cannot replace clinical results, and ample proof of results in chiropractic exists. What is conspicuously omitted from such propaganda charges is that seminars of this kind serve all professions, including medicine and dentistry. It should be pointed out that many business consultant firms are subsidized by medical physicians. It is a thriving industry. The way it works is that a business consultant spends time in the medical doctor's office observing his office procedures. For a fee of about $600.00 he advises the medical doctor on what he can do to increase the volume of his practice, work shorter hours, and make more money.

On the subject of salesmanship, untold millions of dollars are spent annually advertising drugs and creating a drug-oriented society. The medical physician, as the prescriber of these drugs, is the obvious benefactor of this advertising. The next time you turn on the radio or television, count the drug commercials as compared to other products advertised.

THE GREAT HORSE RACE

There is a story of a horse race between two entries, an American and a foreign stallion, that was run on American soil. The American horse won the race and as a result an American newspaper reported the race saying, "A horse race between the great American stallion and the foreign entry had the American entry winning easily."

The foreign newspaper reporting the same race said, "The superiority of our horse breeding was clearly demonstrated in an international horse race today. Although not familiar with the foreign turf, our stallion made a brilliant performance coming in a close second while America's finest entry on familiar soil came in next to last."

This simple story classically illustrates the effectiveness of deceptive reporting without telling an outright lie. The next time you have occasion to hear or read a deceptive propaganda article, just think of the great horse race.

CHAPTER VI

Chiropractic in Medicare

HEW REPORT

IN ENACTING the social security amendments of 1967, the Congress decided it needed more information on the need and the cost of covering licensed independent healing professions such as chiropractic, optometry, and occupational therapy, not included in Medicare.

Congress directed that the study be made by Secretary of Health, Education and Welfare, Wilbur J. Cohen, after a conference committee had rejected a proposal that it be made by the medically oriented United States Public Health Service. Despite the conference committee's rejection, the report "Independent Practitioners Under Medicare," dated December 28, 1968, was prepared within the U.S. Public Health Service, with the results Congress had specifically intended to circumvent—a biased and unreliable report.

The principal device for the preparation of the HEW report was the appointment of two committees, an Ad Hoc consultant group for the independent professions, and an expert review panel for chiropractic. Both of these groups were medically oriented and had professional and institutional bias against chiropractic.

For example, the 22 man Ad Hoc consultant group

included seven medical doctors, one doctor of osteopathy, one hospital administrator, one dentist, one health college dean, and one nursing service official. Of this group, at least 12 were professionally or institutionally prejudiced against chiropractic.

The Ad Hoc group was responsible to Dr. John W. Cashman, Assistant Surgeon General, U.S. Public Health Service, who admitted privately to a representative of the chiropractic profession before the study began, that he was opposed to chiropractic.

During hearings and formation of the study, the Public Health Service rejected repeated requests for chiropractic observers at the meetings of the Ad Hoc consultant group.

The second group, an expert review panel, consisted of eight members. Five were medical doctors and one was a medical school professor. No representation from the chiropractic profession was permitted.

Instead of confining the report to "needs" and "costs" it presented medically biased misstatements of facts about chiropractic, then recommended chiropractic remain excluded from Medicare. Thus, it not only failed to supply Congress with the specific information it requested, but exceeded its authority by ignoring the specific limitations placed upon the study.

THE HEW OCTOPUS

Organized medicine held up this HEW report as "an unbiased, independent government agency report that rejected chiropractic," and relied heavily on it to influence Congress against chiropractic inclusion in Medicare. Furthermore, the report has been used to influence state legislators against chiropractic. Here is the Massachusetts AMA position on the HEW report: "One unexpected beneficial side effect of Medicare may be that it will finally and forever eliminate some of the cults of quackery that continue to thrive. The report to the Congress of former HEW secretary Wilbur Cohen may be the potent weapon needed to eradicate the cult of chiropractic."

The HEW report has been compared to an octopus, with its body in Washington and its tentacles invading the various states. This report has already been used by organized medicine, although unsuccessfully, in at least Massachusetts, New Jersey, Oregon, Iowa, and Illinois in an attempt to eliminate chiropractic.

By October, 1972, the health legislation bill (H.R.1) was near completion. The Senate version of the bill provided for chiropractic health care, while the House version provided for a two year study of chiropractic. Such differences generally are resolved within the House-Senate Conference Committee.

Before the Senate bill went to the Conference Committee, Senator Edward Kennedy introduced an amendment to place chiropractic under another study. In defense of his position, he quoted from the HEW report on chiropractic, repeated the California case of the girl with cancer of the eye, dwelled on the "potential hazard" of denying people proper medical care, and implied that chiropractors generally profess to have a cure-all method of healing. He also repeated the false statement that no scientific evidence exists supporting the validity of chiropractic. But why didn't he first direct these questions and criticisms to either of the two national chiropractic associations?

The Senate, weary and suspicious of another study, and with a number of Senators aggressively voicing support for chiropractic inclusion in Medicare, rejected Kennedy's amendment by a 66–6 vote. Eight other Senators, announced that they, if present and voting, would have rejected the amendment.

The strong Senate support for chiropractic had a significant impact. The House version of the bill gave way to the Senate. The conference committee voted to include chiropractic care in the final bill which was signed into law in October, 1972, to be effective on July 1, 1973.

If Congress had decided against chiropractic inclusion in Medicare for whatever reason, it would have had two significant effects on chiropractic. Organized medicine could have propagated this as "Congress supporting the unbiased HEW report," providing it with an extra weapon in its state and federal drives against chiropractic. With total health care inevitable, medicine could have provided some alternate care to chiropractic at no cost to the patient, posing an economic threat to chiropractic's existence.

The fact that medicine is utilizing spinal manipulation, forming manipulative academies, and teaching week-end spinal manipulative seminars is a known fact. However, a week-end medical manipulator who dabbles in the art of manipulation cannot compare with a chiropractor who studies for years and attains outstanding competency in spinal adjusting.

CHIROPRACTIC COST STUDY IN MEDICARE

The "cost study" for chiropractic inclusion in Medicare was done by the Social Security Administration for HEW. This study was proved grossly inadequate and erroneous. For example, the SSA used a 1965 U.S. Public Health publication entitled *Health Resources Statistics* at a time when a 1968 copy of the same publication was available. The 1965 copy of the publication gave incorrect figures of 23,000 chiropractors in America, while the 1968 issue gave corrected statistics showing 17,000 chiropractors in America. By using the incorrect statistics, the SSA created a false 26 per cent increase in the cost estimate for including chiropractic in Medicare. This error was exposed before the Congressional House Ways and Means Committee by the chiropractic profession in testimony on November 3, 1969.

Why, then, did the SSA use the obsolete publication in its study and create a false cost estimate for chiropractic? The SSA has never answered this question, nor has it withdrawn its fallacious study.

The chiropractic profession provided additional "cost study" statistics before the Ways and Means Committee. These included the figures of 19 of the largest health insurance companies in America, who wrote health insurance premiums totalling $3,879,000,000, or 44 per cent of all the commercial health insurance in the United States. Their overall conclusion was that there was no increase in their costs when they included chiropractic in their health care policies.

Chiropractic, by providing an alternate type of service, removes some patients from costly hospital care and brings them less expensive and possibly more effective care in a chiropractic's office. Since 78 per cent of past costs in Medicare were hospital costs, this is a significant factor in saving taxpayer's money. In addition, it releases many beds in the already overcrowded hospitals.

In 1966, a statistical comparison of chiropractic and medical treatment of back injuries was conducted from the Iowa workmen's compensation records. Conducting the survey was E. Paul Barnhart, a professional consulting actuary from St. Louis, Missouri. His findings were as follows: The average work-time loss per case under chiropractic care was less than one-half of the time-loss under medical care; the average cost under chiropractic care was $68.24 compared to $118.74 under medical care; the average cost of braces and supports under chiropractic care was 81 cents compared to $4.18 under medical care.

The Colorado state compensation department from July 1, 1948, to July 1, 1949, provided figures for a comparative survey of nearly 2,000 patients treated under chiropractic and medical care. The chiropractic patients returned to work in 2.64 days compared to 4.93 days under medical care, or approximately one-half of the time it took under medical care.

In Minnesota, the Associated Insurance Researchers studied 10,000 case files of three major insurance companies, covering a four year period ending in 1957. They found 557 back injury cases. Of these, 281 were handled by medical doctors, 236 were handled by doctors of chiropractic, and 40 were handled by doctors of osteopathy. The average claim under chiropractic was $35.64 compared to $64.60 under medicine.

A 1971 study of statistical information furnished by the Oregon workmen's compensation board, a 24 month study limited to back injury cases involving sprains and strains only, found that the average total cost per case was as follows: Under care of a medical doctor $298.52 average total cost. Under care of a chiropractor $75.92 average total cost.

A 1971 survey of Kansas workmen's compensation records limited to back injury cases involving sprains and strains only, shows average total cost per case as follows: Under care of medical doctor $102.53 average total cost, under care of chiropractor $65.69 average total cost.

Under the California old age security program, records from July, 1962 to June, 1964 reveal that the average cost of chiropractic services was $33.11, compared to an average cost of $76.67 for each of the other health professions. The total number of patients under chiropractic care during this period was 39,253.

In the 1950s, a study of workmen's compensation records of 44 states and Canada, comparing chiropractic and medical treatment cost and wage loss, revealed the following figures: Average cost of chiropractic treatment was $27.07, while the average cost of medical treatment without hospitalization was $50.06, and with hospitalization was $85.34. The wage loss of the average chiropractic patient was $55.42, while the wage loss of the average patient under medical care without hospitalization was $95.06, and with hospitalization was $163.44.

Topped off with the Florida workmen's compensation studies of 19,666 back cases (as discussed in chapter three) in which people under chiropractic care returned to work at one-third the time and cost compared to medicine, the documented examples above are significant factors in light of the fact that back strain costs our economy over one billion dollars annually. Also, the studies support the need for chiropractic in Medicare and all future health programs.

FREEDOM OF CHOICE OF HEALTH CARE

In an unsuccessful drive to keep chiropractic excluded from Medicare, organized medicine frequently repeated the statement: "Chiropractic in its well-financed, never ending political drive for recognition claims people are being denied their freedom of choice in Medicare." Let's examine the second part of that statement first: "People are being denied their freedom of choice in Medicare."

Organized medicine has strongly opposed national health care for many years, referring to it as "the most deadly challenge." In October, 1950, the AMA spent over $3 million for advertising to combat national health care. Covering most leading newspapers, radio and magazines, the popular advertised slogans were: "In America, We Don't Like Compulsion"; "The Voluntary Way is the American Way"; and "When You're Sick, Do You Want Doctors—or Clerks?" National health care was identified with waste, incompetence, and un-Americanism.

Dr. Donovan F. Ward, past president of the AMA, in opposing Medicare likened the AMA opposition to it with Winston Churchill's struggle against the Nazis in 1940 during Britain's darkest hours.

About 90,000 M.D.s were given reproductions of Sir Luke Fildes' painting of a worried doctor keeping vigil by the side of a sick child to be placed in the doctor's waiting room. Under the picture was the caption: "Keep Politics Out of This Picture."

Dr. Edward Annis, president of the American Medical

Association, denounced Medicare as a "hoax and a fraud," and "a step toward the end of democratic government in this country."

The AMA circulated posters and leaflets in opposition to Medicare which said: "The time has come for all of us to stand and be counted on the question of socialized medicine. Your freedom is at stake. Freedom is what we all stand to lose. Your freedom to choose the doctor you believe is best for you." The posters also added, "These freedoms are bound to be lost when the federal government enters the privacy of the examination room, controlling both standards of practice and the choice of practitioner."

Congress responded by introducing into the Medicare Act under Title 18 Section 1801, "Prohibition Against Federal Interference." It also added under Title 18 Section 1802, "Free Choice by Patient Guaranteed." Though this was a written guarantee in the Medicare Act, chiropractic care was denied under this act until 1973. This was a violation of states' rights and a patient's right to choose his own doctor without penalty.

Many examples of the former violations can be cited. In 1973 chiropractic was licensed and regulated in 49 states, the District of Columbia, and Puerto Rico, yet Medicare denied residents of these states the health care approved by the states.

Insurance equality laws had been enacted by the state legislatures of most states, with other states expected to follow. These laws required insurance companies to recognize and pay chiropractic claims on an equal basis with medicine and osteopathy, yet federal Medicare had violated these insurance equality laws and states' rights as guaranteed under Section 1801 of the Medicare Act.

Under Title 19 of the Medicare Act there is a provision for Medicaid. This is a federally subsidized and state-sponsored medical care program for persons under the age of 65 unable to afford medical care. The majority of the states pay for chiropractic care under this Medicaid program.

The indigent person receiving chiropratic care prior to 1973, on being transferred to federal Medicare, had to change his doctor if he expected continued insurance coverage. He had to change doctors in spite of the fact that the doctor of chiropractic may have been familiar with his condition, and that the chiropractic approach to healing may have been the most effective method in relieving his suffering. This was a classic example of violation of the patient's freedom of choice of doctor and his rights in his own state.

It is interesting to observe that the chiropractic profession, which was on record in support of Medicare for senior citizens before it became law, originally was excluded from Medicare while organized medicine, which so violently opposed Medicare, immediately became part of the program.

The hypocrisy of organized medicine was demonstrated when it posed so righteously as the defender of the patient's states' rights and freedom of choice of doctor in its opposition to Medicare. Later, by unsuccessfully campaigning to keep chiropractic out of Medicare, it was perpetuating its hypocrisy by espousing the very violation it once so righteously opposed.

CHAPTER VII

Medicine's Opposition to Medicare

WHAT about some of the reasons the AMA used in its opposition to Medicare? Let's examine them.

In 1961, a group of AMA officers met in Chicago to hear Professor William Demougeot, a professor of speech at North Texas State University, evaluate the AMA's public image and help it in its battle against federal health insurance.

Professor Demougeot assured the medical men that he fully supported their position on federal health insurance. However, he cautioned them against using certain arguments in the presence of knowledgeable people.

First, he agreed that the AMA charge that Medicare would amount to socialized medicine was "a big help in prejudicing the public." He warned the medical doctors, however, to use it in a limited way and never before sophisticated people.

Second, he said the "denial of free choice" was a useful argument, but only to a group not familiar with the facts. He frankly stated that this argument was not true. Professor Demougeot suggested that the best approach was through the statement that Medicare would be compulsory, though he conceded that sociologists and economists could demonstrate that national compulsory health care is justifiable, and cheaper than private health care programs.

Third, the claim that England's medical service was second

rate should not be used in the presence of people acquainted with the system in England. Even though England may have second rate medical care, he insisted, it was much worse prior to its national health program. Moreover, 60 per cent of the doctors and 90 per cent of the patients have been satisfied with the program.

Fourth, he said that the AMA's charge that government health insurance was exorbitant, as opposed to the cost of private plans, was difficult to justify. Why? Because the administrative costs of private health insurance plans ran as high as 25 per cent and were increasing, while England's administrative costs were 12 per cent and going down. He also recommended avoiding discussion about our social security system because its administrative costs were still lower.

Professor Demougeot said that the United States was the only major nation in the world without a compulsory national health system. He added that in 59 nations, no conservative party had ever recommended abolishing such a system. This, in itself, was a potent argument for national health care, an argument the AMA best avoid.

Fifth, he recommended that physicians refrain from using, at least in front of an intelligent opponent, the argument that American medicine was the best in the world because of the free enterprise system and private practice. Improved sanitation, food, clothing, shelter and the patient's ability to pay, all these were important factors in the standard of health and quality of care. He said that numerous countries had higher longevity and lower infant mortality rates, and that all of these countries had national health insurance programs. Furthermore, he reminded them that most medical advances were made by a doctor working on salary, which usually was paid by the government.

In spite of the fact that Professor Demougeot explained these facts to the officers of the AMA, organized medicine had insisted on using these same arguments in its campaign against Medicare.

To complicate an already bad situation, a group of medical physicians wanted to purchase advertising space in the *Journal of the AMA* to present an argument in favor of Medicare. This group was flatly refused! Thus, as the AMA continued its attack against Medicare, it suppressed opposing views of its members.

HEALTH CRISIS

American health care, as compared to its national wealth, is a national disgrace. Senator Edward Kennedy, in his book *In Critical Condition—The Crisis in America's Health Care* wrote: "I am shocked to find that we in America have created a health care system that can be so callous to human suffering, so intent on high salaries and profits, and so unconcerned for the needs of our people. American families, regardless of income, are offered health care of uncertain quality, at inflated prices, and at a time and in a manner and a place more suited to the convenience and profit of the doctor and the hospital than to the needs of the patient.

"Our system especially victimizes Americans whose age, health, or low income leaves them less able to fight their way into the health care system. The health care industry seems by its nature to give more freedom and power to the providers of care, and very little to the people. It is an industry in which there is very little incentive to offer services responsive to the people's needs and demands. It is an industry which strongly protects the profit and rights of the provider, but only weakly protects the healing and rights of the people."

BETTER SPENDING NEEDED

A book entitled, *The American Health Empire*, by Barbara and John Ehrenreich, made some charges which should interest a cost-minded Congress.

According to this book, a group of activists called the

Health Policy Advisory Center (PAC) charge a medical conspiracy exists between hospitals, Blue Cross-Blue Shield, and the medical instrument and drug companies. This is how they say it works.

Most money that pays for health care in the hospitals comes from Blue Cross-Blue Shield, Medicare and Medicaid. The hospitals which get this money control the organizations through a system of "interlocking directorates." Therefore the "Blues" never question the amount of the hospital bills, which means the hospital can raise its fee as much as it wishes, while the hospitals in turn are always ready to support requests for higher medical insurance premium rates by the insurance companies.

PAC goes on to say there is little hope for reform under the present system since it is like pouring large amounts of money into the same leaky jug, resulting in escalating costs without basic improvement.

Pierre de Vise, assistant director of the Hospital Planning Council of Metropolitan Chicago and principal investigator of the Chicago Regional Hospital Study (a project supported by the USPHS), submitted a report which should be especially interesting to taxpayers. The report said: "The challenge for American government is not to spend more, but to spend better, to channel correct annual expenditures of $20 billion into more efficient and accessible delivery systems . . ."

In explaining his position he presented five points:

1. "The federal funding programs essentially subsidize a private for-profit activity that otherwise would go bankrupt.
2. "The physician's reimbursable fee is set neither by actual costs, nor by private market demand, but by a combination of private and public demand. In other words, he charges all the market will bear.
3. "Allowable hospital costs are based on actual costs, rather than on fixed charges. There is no incentive for economy.

On the contrary, the incentive is for physicians to transfer as many of their personnel and equipment costs to hospitals as they can.

4. "Funding programs greatly favor private medical care over group practice or salaried medical care, and inpatient hospital care over outpatient or clinical care, even when the latter are more economical and appropriate.
5. "Public funding programs largely underwrite the private care of the poor and the old, a sector in which private medicine has been scandalously neglectful."

He noted that duplication of special hospital equipment exists, such as for cancer or open heart surgery, and that such equipment is grossly underused. Some south side Chicago hospitals he inspected could handle the needs of cancer patients for the entire state of Illinois. One Chicago hospital inspected had teletherapy equipment (cancer therapy equipment) that had never been used. No one knew how to use it. Proficiency in teletherapy and heart surgery requires frequent practice. Underutilization means rusty skills and possible low quality service. Since general practitioners are reluctant to refer patients to specialists in other hospitals, and hospitals feel they need such equipment for prestige and status without regard to need, costly duplication occurs.

Mr. de Vise said in his report that more and better service at less cost lies in more effective federal cost and utilization control, at least with respect to federally funded programs like Medicaid and Medicare. This, he says, would eliminate unreasonable duplication of costly specialty medical equipment (the cost of which is passed on to the consumer), eliminate any unnecessary hospital inpatient care that could be handled as well with less expensive outpatient care, and reduce abusive practices of physicians charging the federal government "what the market will bear."

He said most of the national health insurance now being considered by Congress "simply proposes to put more money into the present inefficient, wasteful, and top-heavy medical establishment, to perpetuate our failure to match medical capacity to consumer need, to invest scarce resources and manpower in life-threatening conditions, and to neglect the major cause of ill health and death."

In 1971, $80 billion was spent on medical care in the United States. This represented eight per cent of our gross national product. Britain, with a comprehensive health care system, spent only 4.9 per cent of its gross national product for health care.

While European countries spend about five per cent of their gross national product for more comprehensive health care using fewer physicians and fewer hospital beds, we spend eight per cent of our gross national product to give fractional care to a fraction of the people. Furthermore, de Vise estimated that by the late 1970s health care would reach 10 per cent of our gross national product (in spite of President Nixon's price freeze), hospital beds would cost $150 per day, a physician's office call $25, a diagnostic visit $100, and physicians would earn an average of $60,000 a year. If that day should come, he said, there is no doubt that the pressure on government to nationalize hospital and medical services would be overwhelming.

He finally concluded that the big three consumers (federal government, corporations, labor unions) "will come to realize that the United States is the only civilized nation to have its wealth system controlled by private physicians and hospitals, and that the United States is proving to the world that no nation can be rich enough to afford a health system so controlled."

In the same vein, Senator Abraham Ribicoff had this to say: "Medical care, instead of being a public responsibility, is a private business, and is operated more for the convenience of its practitioners than according to the needs of the sick."

Reform in this country is thwarted because it is not

consistent with the vested interest of those groups which control the health system. Organized medicine, the drug corporations, and the insurance companies, all have powerful lobbies. The consumer does not.

ORGANIZED MEDICINE'S REAL REASON FOR OPPOSING MEDICARE

Medicare in 1965 was the first step toward total government controlled health care, which organized medicine fears.

After Medicare became law, Walter Reuther, late president of the United Auto Workers, created a committee of 100 to study and establish a national health insurance program. It was organized labor that helped push Medicare through Congress in 1965 in spite of the strong opposition by organized medicine.

When Gov. Nelson Rockefeller of New York proposed a national health insurance program to all the governors at the 1969 national governors conference, the idea received almost total support.

Currently, many prominent and influential congressmen have dedicated themselves to bringing about total health care in this country. This appears to be the trend for future health care, it is how our leaders are thinking and the direction we are going. Total health care appears to be inevitable within the not too-distant future. It also means that the government will have increasing control of the money to be paid to the physicians, and if there is anything organized medicine fears it is governmental regulation and control of fees.

There have been many news accounts of individual doctors of medicine who, by unscrupulous means, have acquired great wealth through Medicare at the expense of the taxpayer. Such reports can only stimulate Congress to correct such abuses.

A United States subcommittee investigating such abuses in 1969 concluded: "Physicians' fees cannot remain subject to the whims of individual providers of service, if Medicare and Medicaid are to be fiscally predictable and gross abuses are to be stopped."

As time goes on, and especially if any further scandals aggravate the matter, Congress will enact more restrictive and regulatory legislation regarding payments to physicians. Eventually, with total health care insurance and the government in control of the purse strings, medicine will be less profitable to some doctors. The AMA will continue to lose members and influence, weakening its efforts to impose its selfish interest upon the public. Doctors of medicine may some day be relegated into the category of government or civil service employees. Humanitarian motivation, rather than monetary reward, then may attract prospective students into medicine.

Whatever reasons may be offered against national health care by organized medicine, the prime motivator is fear of governmental regulation. Whether organized medicine is justified in its fear is not for discussion here. What we are concerned with is organized medicine's parading under the banner of righteousness and concern for patients while its prime concern is really its financial interest and restraint from governmental control.

CHAPTER VIII

Chiropractic and the National Council of Senior Citizens

ONE of the most scurrilous attacks ever launched against chiropractic came from the January, 1969 issue of the *Senior Citizen News*. The AMA widely circulated reprints of this article, including copies to the members of Congress. Although the article was heralded as coming from a source outside of medicine, a recent disclosure of correspondence between Executive Director William Hutton of the National Council of Senior Citizens and Doyl Taylor of the Department of Investigation of the AMA, revealed that they actually collaborated in the writing of the article.

The article said, among other things, that the "National Council of Senior Citizens, in specific resolutions approved by large majorities of delegates attending its annual conventions, has continued to urge that the services of chiropractors be barred from coverage under the Medicare program." It went on to say, "Since the 1968 convention rejected chiropractors . . ." The article was especially vital because it alleged that the senior citizens, who are the recipients of Medicare, did not want the services of chiropractic.

This newspaper article was a classic example of the use of half-truths, innuendoes, exceptions to the rule, obscure sources, obsolete material, material out of context and fallacious material, as explained in chapter five. It was truly an insult to honesty in reporting.

The above statement regarding the delegates urging that chiropractic be excluded in Medicare is fallacious. Could you imagine a group of properly informed senior citizens voting against their freedom of choice of doctor and for more restrictive health care? It could be compared to a labor union meeting urging less pay and more restrictive benefits for itself.

Based on numerous written statements from some of the most reliable and prominent senior citizens who attended the 1968 convention, here is what really happened there. Though these statements came from many different independent sources, they all corresponded and supported each other. Here is their story.

The Social Security Committee of the 1968 national convention recommended adoption of a resolution urging chiropractic inclusion in Medicare. The proposal for chiropractic was recommended in that committee by Mr. Edward Schroedter, the President of the Allied Councils of Senior Citizens of Wisconsin, and a delegate and member of that committee.

The Executive Committee of the National Council of Senior Citizens did not report out on the floor the Social Security Committee's recommendation for chiropractic inclusion in Medicare, and the Social Security Committee questioned why it was not done. The executive committee gave as its reason the fallacious HEW Ad Hoc Report on chiropractic. Since the delegates were overwhelmingly in favor of the chiropractic issue, and the executive committee (with its medical advisors) was not, it was agreed to do a study on chiropractic and report back the results during the 1969 convention.

Thus the January, 1969 issue of the National Council of Senior Citizens Newspaper published the statement that the delegates rejected chiropractic in Medicare.

With perfect timing, organized medicine had reprints of

that *Senior Citizen News* article circulated to congressmen on the House Ways and Means Committee, just as the committee was deciding on the issue of chiropractic inclusion in Medicare. Although the Senate voted to include chiropractic in Medicare, the chiropractic issue was deadlocked in a tie in the House committee, and before the bill could reach the House-Senate Conference Committee, Congress adjourned for 1970. Of course, the chiropractic bills died and had to be reintroduced in 1971.

POLISH-AMERICAN SENIOR CITIZENS SPEAK OUT

During the 1969 National Convention of Senior Citizens the vice-president of the Polish-American Senior Citizens, Mrs. Eleanor Deka Kiel, who was also a national director of the National Council of Senior Citizens and director of the Chicago Area Councils of Senior Citizens, made several attempts to get the issue of chiropractic brought up for a discussion and delegate vote. Numerous other delegates also tried to get this issue up for a vote. Every effort failed and the executive committee of the National Council of Senior Citizens succeeded in suppressing any discussion or vote on chiropractic, thus violating its 1968 convention agreement.

On November 29, 1969, the vice-president of the Polish-American Senior Citizens wrote a letter to the executive director of the National Council of Senior Citizens, William Hutton, which said:

> I am writing you in regard to the unfair article on chiropractic in the January, 1969 Senior Citizen Newspaper. In my various capacities in senior citizen work, I have spoken to many people and they were all in favor of chiropractic inclusion in Medicare. Your article did not, nor does it, represent the attitude of the senior citizens.
>
> As I was at the 1968 convention, it was obvious to me that the majority of the delegates were for the inclusion of chiropractic in

Medicare. Furthermore, if a vote had been taken at that convention, it was obvious that support for chiropractic inclusion in Medicare would have passed. You quickly pulled out the discussion of chiropractic from the convention, refused delegates to speak in behalf of chiropractic, and submitted it to your biased executive board which committed a great injustice to the senior citizens as they could use chiropractic help.

I am hoping you give serious consideration to my constructive criticism. . . .

This letter was never answered by the national council executive committee!

On December 17, 1969, the vice-president's letter was read and discussed thoroughly at the Polish-American Senior Citizens business meeting. The members at that meeting voted to support her criticism of the national council executive committee by a vote of 148 to 0 and recorded this in their minutes which were mailed to the executive committee. Again, the national executive committee of the National Council of Senior Citizens did not even dignify the Polish-American Senior Citizens with an answer to their protest.

In spite of all the furor raised by the Polish-American Senior Citizens, the medically influenced and prejudiced executive committee of the National Council of Senior Citizens again violated its previous agreement of 1968, and again did not permit discussion or delegate vote on chiropractic during the 1970–71–72 conventions.

Therefore, while the national executive committee exerted every effort to suppress the senior citizen delegates from voting on a chiropractic resolution as recommended by the 1968 national convention social security committee and ignored resolutions for chiropractic inclusion in Medicare from its state senior citizen organizations, it used the *Senior Citizen News* publication to perpetuate fallacious statements about their delegates and chiropractic. At least one state senior citizen organization, even refused membership to the National Council of Senior Citizens until it abolished its prejudiced position on chiropractic.

Meanwhile, organized medicine has frequently quoted the National Council of Senior Citizens as being opposed to chiropractic. This is certainly not a beautiful picture, but nevertheless a true one. The American Association of Retired Persons, with over five million strong, adopted a resolution in support of chiropractic at its convention. Is there any reason to believe that the National Council of Senior Citizens delegates, if given a proper and honest opportunity, would not have done likewise?

Fortunately, Congress was not influenced by the bias of the executive committee of the National Council of Senior Citizens, and voted to include chiropractic in Medicare.

CHAPTER IX

Chiropractic and the AMA

THE AMA has been heavily promoting an antichiropractic propaganda book. It has been urging its members to place copies in their waiting rooms and distribute them to patients. It circulates the book to the news media, radio, T.V., state and federal legislators, libraries, etc. The book, in hard cover and paperback, and which is without a bibliography to support its allegations, relies on the typical propaganda techniques as described in chapter five.

Its author originally wrote on chiropractic in the *National Enquirer*, in a writing style suitable for this tabloid. Examples of earlier *Enquirer* headlines include: "I Cut Out Her Heart and Stomped on it"; "Digs Up Wife's Rotting Corpse and Rips it Apart"; "Kills Son and Feeds Corpse to Pigs."

A former writer for the *Enquirer* noted in *Playboy Magazine*: "How would the words *National Enquirer* look on my resume? Clearly, prospective employees elsewhere in the fourth estate would regard ex-*Enquirer* staffers with disgust and contempt . . .

The writing style of the AMA-supported author has not changed since his article appeared in the *Enquirer*. Nor did it seem to dampen the AMA's enthusiasm for his book.

MEDICAL MONOPOLY

A desire for absolute dictatorial control of the healing arts has been demonstrated by organized medicine, which has violently opposed the inclusion of chiropractic in Medicare. Spokesmen have openly stated in its medical journals that by excluding chiropractic from Medicare, and later from the national health care programs, chiropractic may be eliminated economically—when all other health care is paid by the government. Organized medicine has clearly stated its goal as "the containment and ultimate elimination of chiropractic."

The April 12, 1971, issue of *Medical Economics News* carried an item entitled, "Chiropractors as Physician's Assistants?" Referring to chiropractic it said, "They (chiropractors) might find a place in M.D. offices as physical therapists, according to Dr. James C. MacLaggan, former president of the California Medical Association." He added, "Their manipulative skill could be useful."

The November 15, 1971 issue of the *American Medical News*, a publication of the AMA, revealed a plan of absorbing chiropractors into medicine. In a two-page article largely devoted to chiropractic it stated how doctors of chiropractic had attended nine-month courses at Duke University, and became licensed "physician's assistants." Of course, these doctors of chiropractic had to renounce their independence of medicine, reject their doctor's title, and fall under the total domination of medical physicians.

Thus, while one segment of medicine castigates chiropractic as a worthless cult, the other is admitting its value and is negotiating with chiropractors to obtain "their useful manipulative skill." As a "physician's assistant" however, the chiropractor would be reduced to a humble and obedient servant of the medical physician; chiropractic would cease to exist as an independent healing profession, and medicine would take over and monopolize the manipulative approach to healing.

The American Chiropractic Association expressed its views

of the American Medical Association in a press release in July, 1969. In a four point statement it read:

> **ONE,** that the American Medical Association is an extremist organization that is attempting to use political power to maintain a monopolistic health care situation here in the United States.
>
> **TWO,** that the AMA is more concerned with destroying what they consider "competitive health professions" than they are in cooperating with government and the allied healing fields to get much needed health services to more people at a lower cost.
>
> **THREE,** that the AMA has been using various smoke-screens, including false charges against chiropractic, in order to get the heat off of their record of non support and non cooperation of many public-minded health programs that have been proposed or instituted in the past decade. This includes Medicare.
>
> **FOUR,** that many conscientious medical doctors throughout the country do not support the narrow-minded, selfish and materialistic actions of the American Medical Association—in fact, they are embarrassed by them. Instead, the medical doctor in the field seeks greater cooperation with other health professions, including chiropractic, in order to provide better and broader health service.
>
> It is unfortunate that during a period when our nation is faced with a health crisis, that the AMA does not stop thinking of how it can further its own power and start thinking about how it can help the people. It is indeed a tragedy that so many well-meaning medical doctors are cast as villains because they are represented by an organization that either doesn't know the meaning of, or doesn't practice, the Hippocratic Oath . . . and has forgotten that in America we pride ourselves on personal freedoms, including the freedom of choice to select who will take care of our health problems.

A prominent midwestern congressman has said, and it is in the *Congressional Record*, that the AMA has produced "a record of almost unparalleled opposition to social and economic progress, blindness to need, and resistance to reform."

ANTITRUST ACT VIOLATED

The behavior of organized medicine has resulted in criminal antitrust suits brought against it.

In 1937, a group of federal employees formed a Group Health Association. They hired a number of medical physicians on salary and provided a low cost, nonprofit health insurance plan. Organized medicine opposed this plan, and tried various means to discourage the GHA physicians from continuing the program. Of course, many physicians resigned from the program.

The AMA and the District of Columbia medical society put pressure on the remaining seven physicians who refused to resign from GHA. They were no longer called in for consultations. Patients were not referred to them by other physicians. They also lost privileges at most hospitals in the area.

Just as the seven physicians were about to concede defeat, Thurman Arnold, Chief of the Antitrust Division of the Department of Justice, came to their rescue. The AMA and the District of Columbia Medical Society were indicted for violations of the Sherman Antitrust Act. The government won a unanimous Supreme Court decision, which held that the AMA was guilty of criminal action. The AMA paid the government a $2,500 fine.

ORGANIZED MEDICINE'S QUESTIONABLE BEHAVIOR

Under federal law, the AMA cannot become directly involved in political campaigns without endangering its tax-exempt status. To circumvent this, the AMA formed an independent group for "educational" purposes. It was founded on a $50,000 donation from the AMA. Founded in 1961 primarily to combat Medicare, the new group was entitled the American Medical Political Action Committee (AMPAC).

Within a year after the formation of AMPAC, 46 state medical societies had formed local political committees, which contributed part of their donations and dues to sustain AMPAC.

The directors of AMPAC are carefully selected by the AMA's board of trustees, making AMPAC the political front organization of the AMA.

AMPAC, in its drive against Medicare, has been involved in some questionable dealings. On a dark street corner one night it acquired a recording of an alleged voice of a United Steelworker executive addressing his co-unionists. The voice demanded that funds be collected for use in electing pro-Medicare candidates to Congress. "For those that don't want to give, you shop stewards can always let them know there is still a graveyard shift," the voice said. AMPAC circulated 5,000 copies of this recording to state and county medical societies to stimulate political contributions from medical physicians. The labor executive denied the voice was his, and filed a $400,000 slander suit against AMPAC. Ironically, though AMA claims no control over AMPAC, it printed an apology in its journal and paid $25,000 to the labor executive.

Another example of the questionable standards of organized medicine can be found in the AMA's relation with the tobacco industry. On January 11, 1964, the surgeon general's report was released condemning cigarette smoking. Just before the surgeon general report was made public however, the AMA's chief spokesman, Dr. Edward Annis, addressed the Kentucky delegation. He warned that the report would provide "insurmountable evidence that smoking causes cancer." But he assured them that "the AMA is not opposed to smoking and tobacco, but it is opposed to disease," then went on to assail Medicare. Of course, the AMA insisted that the choice of these two topics in a tobacco-state address was simply coincidental and not intended to enlist the help of tobacco men in fighting Medicare.

Shortly before the surgeon general's report was made public, the AMA had formed a new tobacco research institute.

Immediately following airing of the report, six leading cigarette companies donated $10 million to the institute.

When the House Ways and Means Committee voted on the issue of Medicare in 1964 it was dead-locked in a tie with Congressman John Watts of Kentucky coincidentally reversing his original pro-Medicare position and voting against the issue. This tie assured the defeat of Medicare in 1964.

Shortly afterward, the Federal Trade Commission (FTC) ordered that all cigarette packages and cigarette advertisements must carry a message about the hazards of smoking. The AMA refused to endorse the surgeon general's report and went on record in opposition to the FTC order.

Senator Maurine Neuberger from Oregon said on the floor of the Senate, "I have no way of knowing whether or not the statement by the AMA to the Federal Trade Commission represents the first fruits of this extensive research program. In any event, I find myself growing somewhat apprehensive about the concern of the AMA for the economic well being of the tobacco industry rather than the physical well being of smokers or potential smokers."

The AMA certainly was not representing its members since the *Medical Tribune* reported a survey at that time showing that 95 per cent of the medical physicians thought smoking was harmful to the smoker's health.

In 1968, the AMA's tobacco-subsidized research committee reported in the *Medical Tribune* that the cigarette problem was "far more complex than had been supposed. Many years may be required to gather sufficient facts and data. . . . It is evident that we have a long road to travel and that this will be done slowly."

To assist this "long and slow road" of research into cigarettes, the six tobacco firms gave an additional $8 million to the AMA research group in 1968.

Again in 1969, the House of Representatives while under pressure from the AMA, rejected stronger warnings on cigarette packages.

When the Federal Communications Commission proposed a ban on radio and television cigarette advertising, the AMA went on record as opposing the ban. Dr. Dwight Wilbur, AMA president, said in the *Medical Tribune* of February 17, 1969, that "this is going to require further study by others in government, such as Congress, before any determination can be made."

In spite of AMA opposition, Congress finally agreed on the January 1, 1971, ban on television advertising of cigarettes. It also agreed on the July 1, 1971, deadline for stronger health warnings on a package of cigarettes.

The AMA's policy on drug advertising in its journal is also questionable. Combination antibiotics appeared on the market by 1950. The rationale of combining two or more antibiotics in one pill was that the ingredients would strengthen each other and have a wider spectrum in treating disease. However, an extensive study in 1966 by the National Academy of Sciences—National Research Council (NAS-NRC), under commission of the Food and Drug administration, disproved this theory. It found that the use of combination antibiotics was less effective, irrational, or even dangerous to the patient.

Editorially, the AMA also condemned combination antibiotics as early as 1957. Yet, as late as 1969, and with the results of the National Research Council already made public, the *Journal of the AMA* carried full page advertisements on a combination antibiotic called Panalba. Panalba, which became available in 1961, was one of the 200 most prescribed drugs and was responsible for about $20 million a year in sales for the Upjohn Company. It also became one of the 369 drugs condemned in November, 1970, by the FDA, which ordered it off the market.

The *Journal of the AMA* by carrying ads on drugs gives unofficial endorsement to these drugs. Why did the *JAMA* advertise, and in effect, endorse a drug of a type it had already condemned? Dr. John Adriani, member and former chairman of the AMA Council on Drugs, suggested it could be for the money. To support its undertakings Dr. Adriani explained ". . . the AMA needs every dollar it can get."

Realizing the serious shortcomings of the fixed-combination drugs, NAS-NRC even prepared a "white paper" on their inability to live up to claims made for them, and sent it to the AMA. It was rejected. No reason was given.

Finally, the May 22, 1969, *New England Journal of Medicine*, receiving the white paper, published the findings of the NAS-NRC at about the same time the *JAMA* was running full page ads for Panalba.

The March 5, 1960, issue of the *JAMA* carried a scientific article which documented 36 cases in which baby girls were masculinized by a synthetic hormone taken by their mothers during pregnancy for the purpose of reducing the risk of spontaneous abortion. In spite of this article, the *JAMA* advertised that hormone for months afterwards without one word of warning as to its catastrophic effects.

Senator Gaylord Nelson (D.Wis.), head of a monopoly subcommittee of the Small Business Committee, said during a Senate hearing that an ad for a tranquilizer boasting "environmental depression" was a "massive default of responsibility by the AMA to accept ads that cannot be supported by any scientific claim." He added, "It is most unfortunate when a great profession is perfectly willing to accept an ad that is just plain fraudulent." He warned the AMA to regulate itself before someone else does.

Such is the dismal record of drug advertising in the *JAMA*, a source of advertising which influences the prescription habits of many physicians.

MEDICAL DISSENSION

The *Yale Law Journal* said that a few doctors who are interested in medical politics can easily wield power and influence out of proportion to their numerical strength. It added, "The nominating process, in combination with apathy of the average doctor, assures domination by a single faction within the AMA."

New officers of the AMA usually are elected after being nominated by the nominating committee. The nominating committee consists of those doctors in power, including the president, who are not likely to nominate anyone critical of existing AMA policies. Since electioneering is viewed as ungentlemanly, other nominations are seldom offered from the floor during an election. Thus, liberal or critical physicians have little or no opportunity to attain a voice of authority in the AMA.

Although political influence in medicine is dwindling for the AMA, many physicians still cannot afford to criticize AMA policies. To do so can mean loss of their hospital privileges, denial of referrals and consultations by fellow physicians, or loss of advancement in hospitals or professional appointments.

The medical profession is represented by at least two national organizations, the American Medical Association and the National Medical Association. Although the AMA is the far more vocal of the two and is the greatest spending lobby group in America, neither group speaks officially for the majority of the physicians in America.

State medical societies are eliminating their mandatory memberships to the AMA. The *American Medical News* of May 24, 1971 reported that the Mississippi and Nebraska medical societies voted against mandatory AMA membership of its state members. The new bylaws became effective January 1, 1972. Physicians in New York State in 1971 dropped their mandatory AMA membership requirements for membership in local medical societies. Their universal complaint was that the AMA did not represent them.

This had a significant impact upon the AMA. Of the 344,028 medical physicians in America, 167,272 were dues paying members of the AMA as of December 31, 1970. By

November, 1972, with the above medical societies dropping mandatory AMA membership, the membership dropped to 155,000, or less than half of the nation's medical physicians. Only six state medical societies required AMA membership. They were Arizona, California, Hawaii, Illinois, Oklahoma, and Wisconsin. Feeling the financial squeeze, the AMA had to eliminate numerous councils and committees, lay off staff employees at the AMA headquarters, and raise its membership dues.

Realizing its rejection by state medical societies and its dwindling membership, the AMA house of delegates in 1971 took unprecedented action in an attempt to increase its membership. It voted to allow interns and residents to join the association without requiring membership in a state medical society.

A nationally conducted Harris Poll taken for *Life Magazine* in the latter part of 1970 asked medical doctors if the AMA accurately represented their views in most professional matters. Only 38 per cent answered with an unequivocal "Yes." Thirty-six per cent answered with a positive "No" and the rest gave qualified answers. This is certainly not a record of unity within the medical profession.

Disenchantment with AMA policies has resulted in the formation of the Medical Committee for Human Rights. Consisting of about 7,000 militant medical physicians, with chapters in 30 cities, it regards the AMA as "archaic and irrelevant" and a menace to enlightened medical care. Their disaffection with the AMA is demonstrated by lapel buttons which say: "Caution—The AMA may be hazardous to your health."

Another group, The National Staff Conference, was formed by a group of resident doctors and interns dissatisfied with the way the AMA was representing doctors. Its declared purpose was to form a new national organization. One of its leaders, who viewed the AMA as representative of "entrepreneur medicine," said, "If they don't wake up and listen to the medical men they're headed for trouble. They'll either listen to us, or they'll disintegrate."

Less apparent, but very real, is the growing dissatisfaction within the AMA, with high ranking officials who become critical of the AMA and who threaten to resign. The executive vice-president of the AMA, Ernest B. Howard, acknowledged that criticism from physicians is "causing turmoil in the organization." Morale among the employees at the AMA headquarters also was at an all-time low.

Dr. Joshua Lynfield, a medical physician, wrote in the *American Medical News* December 21, 1970, that the AMA claims to represent its membership without knowing its views. He added, "One does not have to be a prophet to foretell that it is only a question of time before the AMA falls apart."

Patients often identify the AMA with their family medical physician, for whom they generally have a very high regard. Consequently, the AMA has been able to "ride on the coat tails" of such physicians, enhancing its own failing image although often embarrassing the individual physician.

The AMA, well aware of its bleak public image and dwindling membership and income, proposed advertising to regain its stature. The *San Francisco Chronicle* on June 23, 1970, reporting on the 1970 AMA convention, stated that the AMA board of trustees wanted to raise its dues and finance an ambitious $10 million television advertising campaign "to bring credibility to the AMA and pride of belonging to physicians." If the AMA would spend some of the $10 million to set the record straight on chiropractic, and would adopt a policy of professional cooperation with chiropractors, it could go a lot further in advancing its image. When the AMA learns this simple truth it will prosper from it, and all humanity will benefit.

REFORM MOVEMENT WITHIN AMA

Within the headquarters of the American Medical Association is a close knit group of persons who recognize the merit of chiropractic, and are appalled by the antichiropractic activities of their organization. Among these members is a high ranking medical physician who spent over two years compiling evidence against the Department of Investigation of the AMA.

Gathering this information without the AMA's knowledge was no easy task. The AMA headquarters, with its armed guards, security checks, pictured identification tags, closed circuit television surveillance of its employees, and extensive screening of new applicants, made his work hazardous and difficult. The physician released the confidential documents within a book, which he made available to the chiropractic profession, various legislators, labor groups, senior citizen groups, and other concerned persons. His identity was undisclosed so that he could continue to work for reform within the AMA.

The documents revealed that what the AMA was saying publicly against chiropractic was not consistent with what it was saying privately. The book charged that the Department of Investigation of the AMA was guilty of questionable behavior, and that there was a need for Congressional and Internal Revenue investigation of its practices.

In 1975 an alleged former employee of the AMA released numerous confidential documents to the Congressional Committee which prompted federal investigation of AMA for possible postal fraud, illegal campaign contributions, income tax evasion, and violations of the antitrust laws. The anonymous informer was dubbed by the news media as "Sore Throat" after "Deep Throat" of the Watergate scandal.

MEDICINE'S POLITICAL DRIVE

In chapter six we discussed the propaganda statement: "Chiropractic in its well-financed, never ending political drive for recognition claims people are being denied their freedom of choice in Medicare." In examining the charge dealing with chiropractic's political drive, let's examine organized medicine's political drive.

The AMA has the greatest expenditure of any group registered in Washington under the federal lobbying law. The *New York Times* on January 10, 1970, reported that during an election year the AMA and its allies spend about $5 million to get its friends elected and re-elected to Congress. According to some Washington experts, the *Times* said, the AMA is the only organization in this country that could marshal 140 votes in Congress between sundown Friday and noon Monday. The AMA maintains a Washington office with 30 employees, including seven lobbyists, the paper reported.

The *Chicago Sun Times* on March 21, 1971, disclosed that the American Medical Political Action Committee (AMPAC) distributed $700,000 to various candidates in 1970, but that the committee refused to report which candidates received the money.

According to a survey by the *Congressional Record Almanac*, the AMA spent $1,155,935 in 1965 in an unsuccessful campaign to defeat the Medicare bill. This was the third highest expenditure of any lobby group in the history of this country. Who had the first and second highest expenditures in the history of the United States? It was the AMA, of course, in 1949-50, when it fought President Harry Truman's health bill.

The *Congressional Record Almanac* for 1966 provide the following official figures of the 10 highest spending lobbies in 1965.

ORGANIZATION	
1. American Medical Association (this total does not include AMPAC)	$1,155,935.30
2. United Federation of Postal Clerks (AFL-CIO)	175,365.09
3. AFL-CIO (national headquarters)	148,343.61
4. American Legion	139,537.74
5. Committe for Automobile Excise Tax Repeal	116,394.46
6. American Farm Bureau Federation	115,846.00
7. U.S. Savings and Loan League	105,840.20
8. International Assn. of Machinists, District Lodge #44 (AFL-CIO)	104,766.96
9. National Housing Conference Inc.	95,534.40
10. National Farmers Union	87,351.78

The American Medical Association was the highest spending lobby group in 1965, spending more money than the next nine lobbies combined! With its excessive spending to influence Congress, it has been able to impose its influence on the masses of the people in this country.

The above AMA total, however, does not include massive expenditures by AMPAC, the front organization for the AMA. Congressman Cecil R. King of California charged on the floor of the House that organized medicine had actually spent an estimated $7 million in one year, and that there were people who felt that figure was too low.

In 1969, Robert Finch, Secretary of Health, Education and Welfare (HEW), proposed Dr. John Knowles of the Massachusetts General Hospital for appointment as Assistant Secretary of Health, the nation's top health post. The AMA, insisting Dr. Knowles was unacceptable for the post, had Senate minority leader Everett Dirksen carry its message to President Nixon. The AMA exerted such political pressure on the President and the Congress, that Secretary Finch withdrew his nominee. In bitter defeat, Secretary Finch selected Dr. Roger Egeberg, dean of the University of Southern California.

Dr. Richard Lee of the Palo Alto Clinic in California once said, "The AMA is not led by medical leaders, but by medical politicians." We could therefore conclude that an ideal medical politician must place the welfare of his profession first if he wishes to advance politically within it, while an ideal medical physician must place the welfare of the patient first. Reflecting on this thought, it would seem Dr. John Knowles was too much an ideal medical physician to be permitted the nation's highest political health post.

On July 14, 1971, Senator Edward Kennedy of Massachusetts, speaking before his subcommittee on administrative practices, delivered a blistering attack against the AMA. Following are some of his statements:

"No amount of historical gymnastics can hide the public

record of AMA opposition to virtually every major health reform in the last fifty years.

"The organization of our health services is still a shambles. Why? Because the AMA and its friends in political life, and its friends in the health insurance industry have stood in the way of every major step towards an efficient, effective, affordable health care system for the American people.

"Instead of the scientific and public professional organization it was founded as, the AMA has turned into a propaganda organ purveying 'medical politics,' for deceiving the Congress, the people, and the doctors of America themselves.

"The American Medical Association puts the lives and well-being of American citizens below its own special interests in ordering its priorities. It deserves to be ignored, rejected and forgotten."

The AMA responded to the attack by writing a letter to the Democratic Senatorial Fund Raising Committee indicating that Senator Kennedy's position could curtail future political contributions to the party from medical physicians.

Senator Kennedy answered the AMA by repeating some of his previous charges and adding: "The AMA has not sent me or my subcommittee any substantive reply to my statement. Instead, their chief Washington lobbyist has sent what can only be described as a blackmail message to the director of the Democratic Senatorial Campaign committee."

Organized medicine's attack against chiropractic has known no limits. It reached another low during the March 26–28, 1971, model Youth Congress at Lawrence, Long Island. The congress was held at the Lawrence High School and was attended by 300 students from 14 states. It provided them an opportunity to learn the legislative process through actual participation. Some students played the role of representatives while others took the role of senators.

On March 27, one of the representatives introduced a bill to abolish the practice of chiropractic, and to impose a one-to-five year prison sentence on violators. The "congressman" came well-prepared with a suitcase full of antichiropractic literature and a well-planned attack. Without any prior knowledge of the bill, the representatives in opposition were at a disadvantage and unable to provide adequate rebuttal to the statements made against chiropractic. As a result, the bill passed the house.

By an amazing stroke of luck, one of the senators was a daughter of Dr. Julius Dintenfass, a prominent chiropractor and author of the book, *Chiropractic—A Modern Way to Health.* Miss Dintenfass happened to be visiting the house when, to her surprise, the bill to abolish chiropractic was passed.

The following day, the Senate's co-sponsor of this bill requested that the original sponsor from the house be subpoenaed to speak on behalf of the bill in the senate. Again, this congressman repeated his attack against chiropractic. This time the opposition had an opportunity to circulate documented facts about chiropractic and prepared a rebuttal and the senate defeated the bill by a 4 to 1 margin.

Had this bill passed the model congress, you can be sure it would have been sent to Washington to acquaint our congressmen of the views and decisions arrived at by the American Youth Congress.

We could go to even greater lengths discussing the political drives and questionable dealings of organized medicine. But there is already a superb book on the market dealing with this subject, *A Sacred Trust* by Richard Harris. This well-documented book is an absolute must to those wishing to be better informed on organized medicine's political drive.

CHIROPRACTIC'S POLITICAL DRIVE

You have seen organized medicine's political drive. Now, how about chiropractic's political drive?

Dr. J. F. McAndrews, executive director of the International Chiropractors Association, said the association spends approximately 9½ per cent of its annual budget on research and about four per cent of its annual budget for legislative activities. The latter figure includes a Washington legislative representative on less than a full-time basis. Twenty-five per cent of membership dues (of members who joined ICA after July 1, 1972), is given annually by ICA to the member's respective alma mater.

The American Chiropractic Association spends 40 per cent of its total membership dues on its colleges for education, and for research. This is an unprecedented action; no other healing profession does this.

Dr. Louis O. Gearhart, executive director of the American Chiropractic Association, said that the association has spent an average of $35,000 a year for legislative activity in a five year period ending August 1, 1971. This includes one lobbyist at less than a full-time basis. Since the total operating budget has been just under $1 million a year, this means it has been spending approximately four per cent of its budget on legislative activities—a very modest legislative budget, to say the least.

When organized medicine, in the light of its own extravagant lobbying, supports such reference to "chiropractic's well financed political drive," it reduces its charge to the point of being ludicrous.

If organized medicine's lobby is so right and proper, why must it spend so much money to win the support it ought to get solely on merit? It can't say it is spending vast sums out of kindness and generosity, not with its record of opposition to social security for the aged, federal funds to save the lives of mothers and children, old age and unemployment insurance, Medicare, Medicaid, workmen's compensation, the minimum wage law, free chest x-rays, public venereal disease clinics, federal low-interest loans to medical students, child labor laws, veterans benefits, the forty hour work week, extension of social security benefits to the disabled, regional heart, cancer and stroke centers, Red Cross blood banks, Blue Cross, Blue Shield, and compulsory reporting of communicable diseases.

When Congress in 1930 granted federal funds to state health agencies to reduce the death rates in mothers and children, the AMA said it "tended to promote communism."

It opposed group hospitalization insurance plans as "half-baked experiments in changing the nature of medical practice." Incredibly, the AMA even harassed the world famous Mayo Clinic in Rochester, Minnesota, for many years because it was a group practice. In 1932, the *Journal of the AMA* attacked group practice as "medical Soviets."

Dr. Allen M. Butler of the Harvard Medical School summarized the record of the AMA aptly when he said: "In the course of the last few years the AMA has expressed itself on just about everything. And in retrospect they've been wrong every time they've expressed an opinion. Their record is extraordinary."

MONEY CANNOT BUY

Congress, realizing a significant public demand for chiropractic, voted to include it in Medicare in 1973. At least 125 congressmen introduced bills in one year calling for chiropractic inclusion in Medicare. When one congressman was asked his reason for sponsoring such a bill he replied with a simple but powerful statement, "Because my people want it!"

Numerous state federations of labor, representing more than 8½ million persons, a majority of the AFL-CIO membership, gave official support for the inclusion of chiropractic in Medicare.

Every senior citizen organization contacted in the Chicago area regarding chiropractic inclusion in Medicare adopted resolutions for it unanimously.

The Polish-American Senior Citizens, which is headquartered in Chicago, unanimously adopted a resolution for the inclusion of chiropractic in Medicare.

The Chicago Area Council of Senior Citizens Organizations, which represents a total of 76 senior citizen groups and is officially the second largest area council in the United States, also adopted a similar resolution.

The National Association of Retired Civil Employees held its national convention in Buffalo, New York, on June 14–17, 1970. Frank W. Meyer, of Greenfield, Wisconsin, introduced an amendment to the Medicare resolutions which urged that chiropractic be included in Medicare. This amendment was passed without one single objection and became a part of a package of Medicare resolutions which were unanimously adopted. The NARC speaks for about 800,000 retired civil service employees in America today.

Several ethnic organizations adopted resolutions for the inclusion of chiropractic in Medicare. Among these were the Polish-American Congress, the Polish Women's Alliance of America, the German-American National Congress (DANK), and the Czechoslovakian Society of America. The organizations passed their resolutions unanimously.

Official support urging that chiropractic be included in Medicare came also from the Regional Commonwealth of Puerto Rico and the Puerto Rican Congress, which have their home offices in Chicago.

These ethnic organizations officially represent more than 12 million people.

The National Retired Teachers Association—American Association of Retired Persons, is America's largest organization for retired persons. It adopted a resolution urging chiropractic inclusion in Medicare. This organization has a membership in excess of five million.

The Chamber of Commerce of the United States issued a report in 1971 on the nation's health care system. It said, "Freedom of individual choice, both by recipients and suppliers of health care, is a basic human value and an assurance against deterioration in quality or invasion of privacy. . . . The individual American's freedom of choice, to select among all State-licensed health care providers, is an essential attribute of any effective and responsive national health insurance.

By whatever statutory means seems appropriate and necessary, the American health consumer should be guaranteed his right to obtain chiropractic health services and all other licensed health services in any national health insurance program which Congress enacts."

The National Association of Letter Carriers, at their annual convention in 1972, adopted a resolution in behalf of chiropractic in Medicare.

The Brotherhood of Railroad Trainmen, the country's largest railway union, adopted a resolution testifying to the value of chiropractic.

The three and one-half million member Building and Trades department of the AFL-CIO also adopted a unanimous resolution for chiropractic inclusion in Medicare.

The International Brotherhood of Teamsters has given national support for chiropractic inclusion in Medicare.

The Veterans of Foreign Wars adopted a resolution for chiropractic inclusion in Medicare at its 70th national convention in August, 1969. The Disabled American Veterans adopted a resolution at its 1967 national convention for chiropractic in Medicare. The American Legion and Veterans of World War I passed state level resolutions, too.

The United Auto Workers of regions four and five are on record as supporting chiropractic in Medicare.

Organizations representing firemen, policemen, barbers, and tradesmen of every sort adopted resolutions in support of chiropractic in Medicare.

This is the kind of support money cannot buy, and this is just a sample of the support for chiropractic. People from all walks of life appreciate the value of chiropractic from their own experience. People represent the most powerful weapon of all. Finally, the most important qualities that money cannot buy are self-respect, decency, honesty and integrity. These must be earned!

In 1970, the following members of the 91st Congress, sponsored inclusion of chiropractic in Medicare.

SENATE

CONNECTICUT
Abraham A. Ribicoff* (D), Thomas J. Dodd (D)
IDAHO
Frank Church* (D)
INDIANA
Vance Hartke (D)
MONTANA
Lee Metcalf (D)
NEW MEXICO
Clinton Anderson (D), Joseph Montoya* (D)

* *Co-sponsors*

HOUSE OF REPRESENTATIVES

ALABAMA
George Andrews (D), Tom Bevill* (D), William Nichols (D)
ALASKA
Howard Pollock (R)
CALIFORNIA
Glenn Anderson (D), George Brown (D), James C. Corman (D), Don Edwards (D), R. T. Hanna* (D), August F. Hawkins (D), Chet Holifield (D), Harold T. Johnson* (D), R. L. Leggett (D), John J. McFall (D), Thomas Rees* (D), Edward R. Roybal* (D), B. F. Sisk* (D), John V. Tunney* (D), C. M. Teague (R), James B. Utt (R), L. VanDeerlin (D), J. R. Waldie (D), C. H. Wilson (D), James C. Cohelan* (D)
CONNECTICUT
William L. St. Onge (D), Robert N. Giaimo (D)
FLORIDA
Charles E. Bennett (D), J. Herbert Burke (R), William C. Cramer (R), William V. Chappell* (D), J. A. Haley (D), C. D. Pepper (D), Paul G. Rogers (D), Robert L. F. Sikes (D)
GEORGIA
W. S. Stucky (D)
HAWAII
Mrs. Patsy T. Mink (D)
IDAHO
Orval Hansen (R)
ILLINOIS
John B. Anderson (R), Frank Annunzio (D), Harold R. Collier (R), Paul Findley (R), Kenneth Gray (D), John D. Kluczynski (D), William T. Murphy (D), Melvin Price (D), Roman Pucinski (D), George E. Shipley (D)
INDIANA
E. Ross Adair (R), L. H. Hamilton (D), Andrew Jacobs, Jr. (D)
MARYLAND
George H. Fallon (D), Samuel N. Friedel (D), Edward A. Garmatz (D)

MASSACHUSETTS

James J. Burke (D), Harold D. Donohue (D), Thomas O'Neill, Jr. (D), Philip J. Philbin (D)

MICHIGAN

J. J. Conyers (D), Charles C. Diggs (D), Lucien N. Nedzi (D)

MINNESOTA

J. A. Blatnik (D), Joseph E. Karth (D)

MISSOURI

William J. Randall (D)

MONTANA

Arnold Olsen (D)

NEBRASKA

Robert V. Denney (R)

NEW JERSEY

Dominic V. Daniels (D), Mrs. Florence P. Dwyer (R), C. Gallagher (D), Henry Helstoski (D), James J. Howard (D), Joseph G. Minish (D), Edward J. Patten (D), Robert A. Roe (D), Peter Rodino (D), C. W. Sandman (R), William B. Widnall (R)

NEW MEXICO

Ed Foreman (R)

NEW YORK

Joseph P. Adabbo (D), Mario Biaggi (D), Frank J. Brasco (D), Shirley Chisholm (D), Leonard Farbstein (D), Jacob M. Gilbert (D), J. M. Hanley (D), Allard Lowenstein (D), Morton B. McKneally (R), John Murphy (D), Bertram L. Podell (D), Benjamin Rosenthal (D), James H. Scheuer (D)

OHIO

Donald D. Clancy (R), Wayne L. Hays (D), Robert Taft (R)

OREGON

Edith Green (D), Al Ullman (D)

PENNSYLVANIA

Frank Clark (D), John H. Dent (D), Joseph M. Gaydos (D), William J. Green (D), J. P. Vigorito (D), Edward G. Biester (R)

RHODE ISLAND

F. J. St. Germain (D)

SOUTH CAROLINA

W. J. Bryan Dorn (D), John L. McMillan (D), Albert W. Watson (R)

SOUTH DAKOTA

E. Y. Berry (R)

TENNESSEE

John J. Duncan (R), James H. Quillen (R)

TEXAS

Bob Casey (D), Jim Wright (D)

VERMONT

Robert T. Stafford (R)

VIRGINIA

Thomas Downing (D)

WASHINGTON
Brock Adams (D), Thomas S. Foley (D), Floyd V. Hicks (D), Lloyd Meeds (D)
WEST VIRGINIA
Ken Hechler (D)*
WISCONSIN
Alvin E. O'Konski (R)

* *Co-sponsor*

THE DOCTOR SHORTAGE AND THE AMA

The President's National Advisory Commission on Rural Poverty in 1967 reported: "Nowhere in the U.S. is the need for health services so acute, and nowhere is it so inadequate. . . . The scarcity of health manpower and facilities in the low income rural areas is alarming and is not likely to be corrected overnight."

The severe shortage of doctors is often dramatically expressed on billboards along American highways saying, "This Town Needs a Doctor!" The U.S. Public Health Service conservatively estimates our current medical physician shortage in excess of 50,000.

Dr. Alex Gerber, author of *The Gerber Report*, illustrated the situation very well when he wrote: "The problem has passed from serious to drastic, from alarming to critical, and now verges on the disastrous." He added that no responsible authority today questions the need for more doctors; they only ask how many, by what means and how soon they can be provided.

The *Gerber Report* indicates that 5,000 communities in America have no medical doctor at all, and desperately need them. In Illinois, the medical society's placement service had a list of 150 towns in dire need of doctors. Among them was a town of 22,000 population with only one medical doctor, and a six-town trade area without a single medical doctor.

In Effingham, Illinois, in 1970, hundreds of children narrowly escaped exclusion from the "Headstart" program for preschoolers because of a lack of medical doctors to give these children their necessary school entrance health examinations. For many years chiropractors had been legally permitted to give these school examinations. However, in the late 1960s they lost this right through an innocent appearing podiatric school examination bill which was introduced into the state legislature. The bill didn't even mention chiropractic by name. Before the chiropractic profession realized the implication of that bill and could take appropriate measures to amend it, it became law. Legislative efforts to restore the right of chiropractors to give these school examinations were opposed by organized medicine.

In recent years, 20 per cent of the newly licensed medical physicians in the United States have been graduates of foreign universities. Dr. Roimer of the University of California said, "We steal from the rest of the world. We are the only major nation that does not export doctors."

Russia, with 17 per cent more people than the United States, has over 600,000 medical physicians, or about twice as many as the United States. It graduates 28,000 new medical physicians each year. This is about 350 per cent greater than the number of medical doctors graduated annually in the United States.

Russia reportedly sends about 2,000 medical doctors to underdeveloped countries throughout the world every year. We may question the competency of the exported Russian physicians, as compared to the American, but they certainly must bc better than no doctor at all.

When we compare the good will derived from our one hospital ship, *Hope*, we can appreciate the impact the Russian physicians have on the rest of the world. While the Russians are establishing themselves as humanitarians in underdeveloped nations, we are not even able to supply enough medical physicians for our own country. We steal from others. What image do we build for the United States in the Community of Nations?

A primary blame for the shortage of medical physicians must fall squarely upon the American Medical Association.

Offices of medical physicians were empty during the great depression of the 1930s, so the AMA Council on Medical Education advised medical schools to reduce their number of graduates, rather than bring medical care to the millions who were unable to afford it. In 1934, the council's secretary stated: "The time has come when we must still further limit the enrollment of our medical schools." The council, reporting a decrease of 584 future doctors in the class of 1935 said: "This is a most encouraging sign and it is due to the efforts of the Council on Medical Education of the American Medical Association and the Association of American Medical Schools and the Federation of State Medical Boards."

In 1949, the U.S. Public Health Service predicted that by 1960 there would be a shortage of 30,000 physicians. The same year, Senator Lister Hill of Alabama introduced a bill which would have provided more medical schools as well as thousands of medical scholarships to needy students. It passed the Senate but was defeated in the House because of strong AMA opposition.

When President Truman's Magnuson Commission in 1951 correctly forecast a shortage of 45,000 doctors by 1960, the AMA described it as "statistical propaganda" and "intellectual poverty of the commission."

In 1956, President Eisenhower told Congress there was a serious shortage in some of the specialty fields of medicine, and that many rural areas and small towns were in need of physicians. The same year Dr. Dwight H. Murray, who was president of the AMA, reassured the public by saying, "I am confident that we can prove conclusively to the government and to the people of the United States that a sufficient number of physicians is being produced. The extreme predictions of doctor shortages by the alarmists of a few years ago simply have not come true. . . ."

In 1959 the Bane Commission also forecast a shortage of

doctors, urging a 50 per cent increase in the number of medical graduates by 1975. Once again, the AMA rejected that report.

In 1965 Dr. Philip Lee, assistant secretary of Health Education and Welfare (HEW) said, "We need twice as many doctors as we now have." The same year Dr. John C. Nunemaker, then assistant secretary of the AMA's Council on Medical Education, still insisted, "There is a tremendous demand for more doctors, just as there is for luxurious cars and yachts. But we can't show there's an actual shortage, especially as compared with the rest of the world."

Finally, in 1966 the AMA realized its shortsighted attitude and reversed its position on the need for more doctors. Tragically, it came too late. Congress, now involved with Vietnam and in an economic bind, did not see its way clear to providing the necessary aid for more medical schools.

In a solemn and ironic note, it was recently estimated by Pierre de Vise of the Metropolitan Hospital Planning Council that 1,000 persons die each year for want of medical care in the city of Chicago, the city in which the AMA has its headquarters.

DECEPTIVE PRACTICES OF THE AMA

Physical Culture Magazine, which was published by Bernarr MacFadden, ran a six month series of articles on the AMA beginning with the December 1926 issue. It showed how the AMA and state medical societies were politically motivated and created medical monopolies under the guise of acting in the public interest. It showed how it used its code of ethics as a "public be damned" conspiracy, and harassed those medical doctors not complying with its dictates. The ancient exposé reveals that the AMA has not "degenerated" into a political propaganda machine as some of its critics will say; its policies *always were* degenerate. It reflects the wisdom of Will Rogers when he said, "Things ain't like they used to be . . . and probably never was."

CHAPTER X

Chiropractic and Medical Education

MEDICAL EDUCATION

IN THE past century as many as 460 medical schools existed in America. Most of them were, by all standards, even those applied in the late 19th century, grossly inadequate. Most of them closed, not because of their inadequacies, but because they were poor business ventures.

By 1900, about 160 medical schools remained and fewer than six of these required any college preparation. Of all the medical schools in existence, Johns Hopkins and Harvard were considered the only adequate institutions of the time.

The Carnegie Foundation, concerned with the bleak conditions of medical learning, retained the renowned educator, Dr. Abraham Flexner, to make a study of these medical schools. He was a doctor of education, not of medicine, and was unbiased in his opinions.

Dr. Flexner personally visited 147 American and seven Canadian schools. His report, *Medical Education in the United States and Canada*, was published in 1910; it labeled the medical schools as disgraceful and shameful. Flexner concluded that only 31 of the existing 155 medical schools deserved to exist. The rest he considered fly-by-night diploma mills which extracted tuitions from unqualified youths, offered inferior medical courses, and issued medical degrees.

His powerfully written and uncompromising report attracted national attention. The reaction of the medical schools toward Dr. Flexner was vicious. He was threatened with law suits, and threats were made against his life. Nevertheless, the Flexner report was the catalyst for a revolution in the medical world.

Dr. Flexner submitted reports on the various medical schools he visited. The city of Chicago, in respect to the medical education of its 14 schools, was called "the plague spot of the country." Dr. Flexner explained that the state law was fairly adequate, for it empowered the board of health to establish a standard of preliminary education, laboratory equipment, and clinical facilities, thus fixing the conditions which entitled a school to be considered reputable. He added, "With the indubitable connivance of the state board, these provisions are, and have long been, flagrantly violated. Of the 14 undergraduate medical schools above described, the majority exist and prepare candidates for the Illinois state board examinations in unmistakable contravention of the law and the state board rules."

Writing about one medical college in Oakland, California, he said: "Its so-called equipment is dirty and disorderly beyond description. Its outfit in anatomy consists of a small box of bones and the dried-up filthy fragments of a single cadaver. A few bottles of reagents constitute the chemical laboratory. A cold and rusty incubator, a single microscope, and a few unlabeled wet specimens, etc., form the so-called 'equipment' for pathology and bacteriology. . . . The school is a disgrace to the state whose laws permit its existence."

The physiology lab of one medical school consisted of nothing more than one blood pressure instrument. Another medical school had signs "Anatomy" and "Physiology" on doors, which were conveniently locked and the keys unavailable. Returning to the school at night, Dr. Flexner bribed the janitor to open the rooms. He found them devoid of equipment.

The Brooklyn Postgraduate Medical School had "no teaching facilities worth mentioning" and was "a reproach to the state." The University of Denver's medical school had "a few cases of books in the office behind the counter." The University of Buffalo medical department had "no dispensary records worthy the name." The San Francisco Hahnemann school had no experimental physiology because "the instructor doesn't believe in it."

Referring to the medical schools in Los Angeles, Kansas City (Kansas), St. Louis, Lincoln (Nebraska), Cincinnati, New York City, and two at Atlanta, Dr. Flexner said: "None of the schools has anything remotely resembling the laboratory equipment which all claim in their catalogues . . . The Hospital School at Atlanta, starting on four weeks' notice had time to get students, but not to get means of teaching them . . . The remaining five eclectic schools are without exception filthy and almost bare. They have at best grimy little laboratories for elementary chemistry, a few microscopes, some bottles containing discolored and unlabeled pathological material, an incubator out of commission, and a horrid dissecting-room, when dissecting is in progress. The St. Louis school was the proud possessor of some new physiological apparatus . . . but there was no place to use it and no sign of its use . . . The other Atlanta, the Los Angeles, and the Lincoln schools have even less . . . Of the eight schools under discussion, none has decent clinical opportunities . . . The eclectics are drug mad; yet with the exception of the Cincinnati and New York schools, none can do justice to its own creed. For they are not equipped to teach the drugs or the drug therapy which constitutes their sole reason for existence."

Referring to the Hering (Chicago), Southwestern, Pulte, Atlantic, Detroit, Kansas City schools he said: "Six schools remain—all utterly hopeless: Hering, because it is without plant or resources; the other five, because in addition to having nothing, their condition indicates the total unfitness of their managers for any sort of educational responsibility. The buildings are filthy and neglected. At Louisville no branch is properly equipped; in one room, the outfit is limited to a dirty and tattered manikin; in another, a single guinea pig awaits his fate in a cage. At Detroit the dean and secretary "have offices downtown"; the so-called laboratories are in utter confusion. At Kansas similar disorder prevails. At the Atlantic Medical appearances are equally bad."

Dr. Flexner noted: "The advertising methods of the commercially successful schools are amazing . . . One offers any graduate who shall have been in attendance three years a European trip." He wrote: "Not infrequently advertising costs more than laboratories. The school catalogues abound in exaggerations, misstatements, and half-truths." For example, the Halifax Medical College boasted: "First-class laboratory accommodation is provided for histology, bacteriology and practical pathology." Dr. Flexner found "one utterly wretched room" was provided for all three.

At one school Dr. Flexner was told: "It is idle to talk of real laboratory work for students so ignorant and clumsy. Many of them, gotten through advertising, would make better farmers. There's no use in having apparatus for experimental physiology—the men couldn't use it: they're all thumbs."

On scholastic requirements of the schools Dr. Flexner wrote: "Many of the schools accept students from the grammar schools. Credentials, if presented, are casually regarded and then usually returned; a few may be found, rolled up in a rubber band, in a dirty pigeonhole. There is no protection against fraud or forgery."

At the medical department of the University of Georgia, Dr. Flexner was told: "We go a long way on faith." In visits to medical colleges, Dr. Flexner found certificates from nonexistent schools as well as from nonexistent places.

Regarding school entrance examinations he wrote: "Low entrance examinations flourish, then, for the benefit of the poor school, not of the poor boy."

Remarking on the courses of study of medical students, Dr.

Flexner said: "The low grade southern schools have a nominal seven month's course; but they allow students to enter without penalty several weeks later and have liberal Christian holidays besides, the course is actually less than six months."

Thus, in 1910 it was a simple task to falsify some school records which the existing medical schools would accept without question, take less than six months of inferior training and receive a diploma to treat the sick. Such was the plight of the medical schools not too many years ago, and youthful graduates of that era can still be in practice today.

A dean of a southern medical school wrote: "We will advance to the highest possible requirements just as soon as the conditions will admit, and we are ready now to open next session under highest requirements if the wherewith to pay expenses is in sight." Dr. Flexner observed that the above statement was simply a question of college survival.

Indeed, the "wherewith to pay expenses" and financial assistance came to the medical schools. Dr. Flexner's report aroused such great public concern that the Rockefeller, Eastman, Rosenwald and Harkness Foundations contributed $200 million to upgrade medical shools. Even so, by 1920 almost half of the medical schools had closed their doors.

The *JAMA* in 1965 stated that the last of the unqualified medical schools had finally disappeared—a $200 million donation, millions of dollars annually from the federal government, and fifty years later! Thus, uniform good medical education in the United States is a comparatively recent development.

One myth about educational standards of medical schools today is that medical students are predominantly "A" students. The inference is that all medical doctors were brilliant students. This is far from the case. A study of five typical medical shools revealed that 12 percent of the medical students were "A" students in undergraduate school. Twelve per cent were "C" students, and the majority—76 per cent—were "B" students.

The *JAMA* of November 25, 1968, stated: "Many persons, including some doctors, seem to believe that medical schools predominantly accept 'A' students and that the 'C' student has no chance of acceptance. Through the years for which records are available, this is simply not true. Nor is there any evidence that schools generally have raised or lowered their requirements."

The facts presented here are not intended to demean any senior medical physicians of today who might have been graduated around 1910-20 or so. Their years of professional experience should certainly qualify them by now. Nor is it intended to demean the more contemporary medical graduates. It is done, rather, to present the whole story of the conditions that have existed in the healing professions, providing the seamy side the medical propagandists conspicuously avoid while making critical references to chiropractic's earlier education.

CHIROPRACTIC EDUCATION

Chiropractic education has been undergong its own 'Flexnerian Revolution.' The Saunders and Badger Reports, released in 1958 and 1960, outlined the necessary measures that chiropractic should take for professional advancement. Unlike the Flexner report, they were obtained and paid for by the chiropractic profession itself. The reports emphasized the need for the highest possible educational standards in its colleges.

The chiropractic leaders supporting more stringent college requirements felt that some colleges were dragging their feet. Other chiropractic leaders believed that some of these goals were excessive, self-destructive and unrealistic in the light of medical propaganda, public ignorance, and governmental neglect. They asked, "If we did all these things, would the foundations and federal government finally become concerned and support chiropractic colleges as they do the medical schools? Would the AMA guarantee it would cease its relentless drive to eliminate chiropractic and instead adopt a policy of mutual cooperation? Would HEW abandon its medically prejudiced attitude toward chiropractic?"

In spite of such adverse circumstances, 86.8 per cent of 6,000 chiropractors polled by Batten and Associates in 1962 said that the standard of chiropractic education must be brought to a level which will qualify the colleges for federal approval of their accrediting agency. Of the others, 10.4 per cent had no answer or opinion, and 2.8 per cent saw no reason for obtaining federally approved accreditation.

Some chiropractic colleges have merged in an effort to strengthen their schools. An all-out effort is being exerted by the chiropractic profession toward the highest possible educational standards. Even organized medicine, though it publicly criticizes chiropractic education, privately concedes that chiropractic colleges have made significant strides in the field of education.

The chiropractic profession had founded the Association of Chiropractic Colleges and the Council on Chiropractic Education. Both were autonomous national organizations advocating high standards of quality in chiropractic education. They established criteria of institutional excellence, evaluating and accredited chiropractic colleges through accrediting commissions, and publishing lists of those institutions which conform to these standards and policies.

Commissions on accreditation conducted field inspections of all colleges. The results were reported to the accrediting agencies and classifications of these colleges were made public.

Both agencies were patterned after the federally recognized councils in allied professions, including optometry, podiatry and osteopathy. They established criteria for accrediatation. A few of these are as follows:

1.) Each college should be incorporated as a nonprofit institution with control vested in a board of trustees, composed of chiropractors and public spirited men and women receiving no financial benefits from the operation of the college.

Furthermore, none of the assets or income should benefit anyone.

2.) Each college should use uniform accounting procedures to conform as far as possible with the reporting methods of the U.S. Office of Education.

3.) Colleges should permit authorized persons to inspect facilities, interview faculty members and administrators, study finanacial and corporate records, and examine student credentials.

4.) Each college faculty should consist of graduates of recognized colleges of the arts and sciences. All basic science instructors should have at least a bachelor's degree in the basic sciences.

5.) All faculty members should have graduate or postgraduate training and clinical experience in the field they teach.

6.) The colleges should have adequate physical facilities and maintain laboratories for practical work in anatomy, histology, physiology, chemistry, histopathology, clinical pathology, bacteriology, roentgenology, and chiropractic technique.

7.) Each college should have an affiliated clinic under strict supervision of the college, for training the extern in proper patient care and management.

8.) Each college should have teaching aids and equipment for classroom demonstration, a museum containing an adequate collection of normal and pathological specimens labeled and catalogued, and an adequate library under charge of a trained librarian.

9.) An acceptable college cannot derive its income solely from students' fees, but must show adequate additional income.

10.) The college curriculum shall not be less than eight semesters. The minimum course shall consist of 4,200 hours.

High educational standards in chiropractic is supported by the National State Presidents' Congress which adopted a resolution urging all chiropractic colleges to require two years of college credit as a prerequisite. The congress has the bipartizan support of virtually every state chiropractic organization in America. Both chiropractic accrediting agencies supported the two-year extra professional college requirement of its colleges.

The accrediting agencies introduced such stringent criteria in spite of being a profession disparaged by medical propaganda, spiraling costs and public ignorance, and plagued with indifference and neglect by the same foundations and federal government which poured millions of dollars into medical schools and research.

Chiropractors agree in most areas of discussion. They usually have the best interests for chiropractic in mind and want to see chiropractic enjoy the finest possible standards. They agree that the foundations and federal government should be aroused to greater interest in and concern for the chiropractic colleges and chiropractic research. They agree that chiropractic education and research should be supplemented by federal assistance, and that the people would be the ultimate beneficiaries of the finest possible care. Finally, they all agree that health care cannot be considered the finest unless it utilizes all available resources, which includes chiropractic.

U.S. OFFICE OF EDUCATION

As previously mentioned, the chiropractic profession had two of its own accrediting agencies, the Association of Chiropractic Colleges and the Council on Chiropractic Education.

The chiropractic profession, in an effort to accredit one of its agencies, met with representatives of the U.S. Office of Education. Of course, the Office of Education only could accredit one agency within a profession.

The nursing profession once was faced with a similar situation. One of its accrediting agencies was supported by the American Nurses Association while the other was supported by the National League for Nursing. Each agency, of course, felt it should become the federally recognized accrediting agency for nursing.

Realizing the situation that existed, the U.S. Office of Education took the initiative with the nursing profession, and helped them form an accrediting agency for both organizations—then approved that agency.

The Office of Education took the same initiative with chiropractic in helping it get one agency approved. The CCE became approved August 24, 1974.

Of course, the Office of Education is part of HEW, and one of its sister agencies in HEW is the U.S. Public Health Service, which has demonstrated its bias with its fallacious Ad Hoc report on chiropractic. But we had a right to expect independent professional judgment from the U.S. Office of Education.

The purpose of accreditation is to upgrade the educational process and to protect the public interest. Whether or not the chiropractic colleges had an officially approved accrediting agency, they would have continued their educational programs. From the viewpoint of the public interest it did not make sense to keep the chiropractic colleges in the educational doghouse. It far better serves the millions of chiropractic patients to have an officially approved accrediting agency which can, with official sanction, help further to upgrade the chiropractic colleges and thus better to serve the public interest.

Other professional schools, especially in the health field, have received millions in federal grants, contracts, and other forms of financial aid. Chiropractic colleges had been unjustly denied all this, yet they have done a superb job of educating an important segment among the health professions. Was it asking too much to urge the foundations, federal government, and especially the Office of Education to express the same interest, concern, initiative, and support for chiropractic colleges as for nursing schools? Certainly not.

A chiropractic spokesman once said, "It took the medical schools $200 million in grants and 50 years to upgrade their education, and that does not include the millions of dollars they received annually from the federal government. If the chiropractic colleges could receive a fraction of the financial support going to the medical schools, it would have a profound effect upon their educational program."

The cost of building and maintaining chiropractic colleges is small compared to the cost of medical schools. For example, the new Penn State Medical School began with a $50 million gift from the Milton S. Hershey Foundation, and it is already receiving additional support from the state. The cost of the Mount Sinai School in New York is approximately $100 million. Thus, building a new medical college can cost an enormous $100 million—by conservative estimate. For a mere fraction of that amount, the federal government could not only upgrade every single chiropractic college in this country, but adequately subsidize them for many years. To do so would provide our citizens with the most sophisticated chiropractic health care possible.

The following is a 1976 list of all the chiropractic educational institutions in the United States, Canada and Europe:

Canadian Memorial Chiropractic College
1900 Bayview Ave., Toronto, Ontario, Canada, M4G3E6
Cleveland Chiropractic College
3724 Troost Avenue, Kansas City, Missouri, 64109
Cleveland Chiropractic College
3511 West Olympic, Los Angeles, California, 90019
Columbia Institute of Chiropractic
255 Valentine Lane, Old Brookville, N.Y., 11545
Life Chiropractic College
1269 Barclay Circle, Marietta, Georgia, 30062
Logan Basic College of Chiropractic
430 Schoettler Rd. Chesterfield, Missouri, 63017
Los Angeles College of Chiropractic
920 East Broadway, Glendale, California.
National—Lincoln Chiropractic College
200 East Roosevelt Road, Lombard, Illinois, 60148

Northwestern College of Chiropractic
1834 S. Mississippi River Blvd., St. Paul, Minnesota, 55116
Palmer College of Chiropractic
1000 Brady Street, Davenport, Iowa, 52803
Pasadena Chiropractic College
774 E. Green St., Pasadena, California, 91101
Sherman College of Chiropractic
Box 5502, Springfield Rd., Spartanburg, South Carolina, 29301
Texas Chiropractic College
5912 Spencer Hwy, Pasadena, Texas, 77505
Western States Chiropractic College
2900 N.E. 132 Avenue, Portland, Oregon, 97230
International Chiropractic College
Sonora House, 300 Little Collins, Melbourne, Australia
Anglo-European College
2 Cavendish Road, Bournemouthe, BHIRA, Hampshire, England

CHAPTER XI

Heretical Giants

HISTORICALLY, many of the greatest contributors to the healing arts, and to humanity, have been victims of unbelievable intolerance, ignorance, hatred and persecution. Today they are acclaimed as great heroes. Books are written about them, monuments and statues have been erected for them, and a world without their contributions would indeed suffer a great loss.

In this chapter, we will meet some of these courageous men and women in the healing arts.

PARACELSUS

In the early 1500s, a Swiss alchemist and physician, Philippus Bombastus von Hohenheim, considered himself greater than the renowned Roman philosopher and medical scholar called Aurelius Celsus, with whom he was frequently compared. Accordingly, he named himself "Paracelsus."

Highly critical of the medieval philosophies of healing in his time, he recommended that the books of Galen and other ancient healers be publically burned as a symbol of their worthless and erroneous teachings. This he personally did at night, surrounded by his followers, while proclaiming, "So the flames of a dying dogma can be seen by the Pope in his chambers."

In Basel, when a famous printer by the name of Frobenius suffered with severe ankle and foot pains, his physicians recommended amputation. Turning to Paracelsus for help, he was treated with chemicals and tissue manipulation. The patient recovered, and the cure was proclaimed far and wide; it was most likely accomplished by the manipulation.

Paracelsus was an itinerant physician traveling throughout many countries and healing many people along the way. His ability as a physician earned him the admiration and gratitude of many patients, but his outspoken ways earned for him the hatred of physicians wherever he went.

His contribution to healing was monumental. He is credited with revolutionizing the science of chemistry and pharmacy and with advancing medicine from the medieval to the renaissance era.

Although his contributions to healing were very significant, he was subjected to so many merciless attacks by his fellow physicians that the word "bombastic" originated from his name. Webster's dictionary today defines bombastic as "high sounding, but unimportant or silly language of little substance."

He died at the age of 48. The cause of his death is not certain, though it is generally believed to have been at the hands of his medical enemies.

In Basel, Switzerland, there stands a statue in memory of this hero for his great contribution to healing.

MICHAEL SERVETUS

Michael Servetus was a Spanish physician and theologian living in the early 16th century. His contribution to healing was to expose the erroneous concept of human blood circulation and to introduce his new concept of pulmonary circulation.

The clergy, suspecting he used human cadavers to disprove Galen's theory, regarded this as blasphemy. He also angered the physicians because he dared to disprove an old, established falsehood and advance a new idea on circulation of blood through the lungs.

His unpopularity with his fellow physicians and the clergy, including the powerful Christian leader, John Calvin, resulted in his being tied to the stake and burned to death.

ANDREAS VESALIUS

Andreas Vesalius (1514–1564) was an anatomist who dissected human cadavers in an effort to learn the secrets of life. He uncovered many errors taught in anatomy for 1,400 years by the followers of the unquestioned authority of the time, Claudius Galen. He showed with overwhelming proof that 50 per cent of Galen's information was in error. Galen never saw the inside of a human body; his research involved dissecting animals and applying his knowledge of anatomy to human beings.

In spite of the fact that Galen never saw the inside of a human body, and Vesalius personally dissected 1,000 human cadavers over a period of 32 years, Vesalius' colleagues blindly rejected his teachings. In fact, his fellow physicians demanded he be severely punished for disturbing God's dead. The appropriate punishment for such a crime was death at the stake.

Vesalius became despondent, frightened and bitter. He burned his life's work of 32 years including his manuscripts and the finest anatomy charts the world had ever known. Finally, he fled in fear of his life.

He took refuge with King Charles V, becoming his private physician, but to no avail. As the demands for his punishment became more vocal, the King compromised by sending Vesalius to the Holy Land to "repent for his sins." On returning from the Holy Land he was shipwrecked on a small island where his body was later found.

Thus ended the life of one of the world's greatest anatomists. Completely rejected, he met death, loneliness and despair. His greatest crime was to expose the institutionalized falsehoods that his fellow physicians had so fanatically espoused for 1,400 years.

WILLIAM HARVEY

William Harvey, an English physician, was born in 1578. His contribution was to accurately describe the flow of blood in the human body and disprove the existing false theories of that time. Through exhaustive vivisection on at least 40 different species of live animals, Harvey was able to demonstrate that the flow of blood begins at the left ventricle of the heart, makes a large circle of the body, and eventually returns to the heart by way of the vena cava. He demonstrated that the heart was a muscular organ which pumps the blood. He also introduced the doctrine of pulmonary circulation, insisting that the blood passed through the lungs on the way back to the heart.

His doctrine was criticized and condemned by his fellow physicians. While he was away from home his laboratory was invaded and all his manuscripts and medical specimens were destroyed or plundered.

Although his teaching was mercilessly attacked for many years, he was a man of quiet conviction and moderate in his criticism of his critics. Living to the age of 80, he was fortunate enough to see his doctrine become recognized during his lifetime.

GEORGE BODINGTON

The idea of sanatoria for the treatment of tuberculosis was first proposed by Dr. Bodington in England in 1840.

He wrote an article on tuberculosis with a very formidable title, "An Essay on the Treatment and Cure of Consumption on Principles Rational and Successful with Suggestions for an Improved Plan of Treatment of the Disease among the Lower Classes, and a Relation of Several Successive Cases Restored from the Last Stages of Consumption to a Good State of Health."

The title was not as formidable as the reaction to it by his colleagues. He met the same fate as the other pioneers of a new idea. His ideas of fresh air and good nutrition were completely rejected, and he was attacked and ridiculed by his contemporaries.

His disappointment was reflected in a letter to his son many years later in which he said, "I often think that when I am dead and buried perhaps the profession will be more disposed to do me justice than whilst I live."

The first sanatorium for tuberculosis was not established in England but in Germany by Dr. Herman Brehmer in 1859. Dr. Bodington's prescient letter to his son proved to be accurate.

IGNAZ SEMMELWEIS

Ignaz Semmelweis was a Hungarian physician and obstetrician born in 1818. Early in his career at the Vienna General Hospital in Austria, Semmelweis discovered the cause of the dreaded childbed or puerperic fever.

Whenever a pregnant woman died her corpse was wheeled into the autopsy room and within 24 hours an autopsy would be performed on her by the obstetricians and students. Afterwards, the same physicians would go to the maternity wards and perform pelvic examinations on the living women using their bare and contaminated hands. Semmelweis observed that it was the women who were examined by the contaminated teachers and students who became sick and died. He documented devastating statistics which should have convinced even the most stubborn minds, but to no avail.

Semmelweis found that women in labor were laid upon filthy sheets which actually stank of decomposed blood and uterine discharge. He urged his fellow physicians to practice proper hygienic measures with themselves, their patients and their environment. He insisted that they properly wash their hands before examining pregnant women. The obstetricians, vainly wishing to maintain a good image for their patients, preferred to wear blood spattered gowns. They felt that a clean gown meant that he was not as busy—consequently not as good a doctor.

In spite of the fact that Semmelweis brought the mortality rate down from 16 per cent to just over one per cent at the Vienna Hospital while he was there, the lowest death rate in the history of the hospital, he was viewed with disbelief, hatred and contempt by lazy students, prejudiced colleagues and jealous superiors. His annual contract with the hospital was not renewed and he found himself friendless and without work.

His successor threw away the wash basins and the mortality rate among child bearing women again returned to an alarmingly high level. In spite of all this, the doctors still rejected the by-now obvious truth.

Unable to get work in Vienna, Semmelweis returned to Pest, Hungary, and took charge of a small lying-in hospital. He continued to practice and teach his doctrine, only to meet the same disbelief and rejection. When he published the book, *The Etiology, the Concept, and the Prophylaxis of Childbed-Fever,* which provided overwhelming proof of his doctrine, Semmelweis provoked even greater hostility from his medical colleagues. A sensitive and compassionate man, he suffered great mental anguish as he saw and heard the dying groans of young women, and the orphaned or dying children they bore.

The fateful toll of bells ringing through the night signaling the coming of the priest to give the sacrament to the dying mothers also added to his torment. Semmelweis wrote, "Even to me myself it had a strange effect upon my nerves when I heard the bells hurried past my door; a sigh would escape my heart for the victim that once more was claimed by an unknown power. This bell was a painful exhortation to me to search for this unknown cause with all my might. . . . without difficulty it was arranged that for the future the priests would take a roundabout route, without ringing the bell, so as to reach the sick-chamber in silence and unobserved."

Unable to endure his mental torture he was driven to insanity and was admitted to a mental asylum in Vienna, where he died in 1865 of an infection resulting from the illness he dedicated his life to eradicate. He was buried in an obscure grave.

Soon after Semmelweis left the Pest Hospital, the maternity death rate again reached alarmingly high proportions and still the physicians blindly rejected his doctrine.

Eventually, Dr. Semmelweis was exonerated and suddenly Hungary, Germany and Austria all claimed his body, insisting he was their native son. Amidst international protest, his body was removed from Vienna and taken to Budapest.

In 1906, a monument was erected in Budapest in honor of Hungary's greatest physician of all time, one of the world's greatest pioneers in surgical asepsis. A book based on Dr. Semmelweis' life entitled, *The Cry and the Covenant*, by Morton Thompson, became a best seller. It is the deeply moving and tragic story of a totally dedicated man, of his love and compassion for humanity, and of his frustration and despair.

LOUIS PASTEUR

Louis Pasteur lived from 1822 to 1895. A very popular theory during his time was called "spontaneous generation," which insisted that organisms could originate in nonliving matter independently of other living matter. When Pasteur disagreed with the century old theory he became subject to scorn and ridicule. Pasteur insisted that pathogenic organisms could not be created within a sterile container, but that the entrance often was gained through germ laden dust in the air.

When his battle with the physicians and surgeons was at its height, he received a letter from Dr. Joseph Lister, who told him how his work had influenced his own thinking on surgical procedures.

Eventually, Pasteur proved he was correct, and many honors were bestowed upon him. He was called "the most perfect man ever to enter the kingdom of science," and was named the "Father of Bacteriology."

On December 27, 1892, men gathered from every corner of the world to honor him. Too weak to address the assembly, he had his son read his address. One of his closing statements said, "Young men, young men, whatever your profession may be, do not let yourself be touched by barren skepticism, nor discouraged by the sorrows of certain hours that pass over a nation."

Lister, who had come to pay tribute to his master, stood up and embraced him. As they stood in this symbol of common brotherhood of science, each man realized, perhaps better than anyone in the audience, the true meaning of Pasteur's closing words.

JOSEPH LISTER

Lord Joseph Lister lived from 1827 to 1912. He advocated absolute cleanliness of the physician: the hands, the instruments, the incision, and the bandages. Although he was subjected to ridicule and condemnation because of his views, he continued his research with antiseptics. Incredibly, his colleagues insisted that pus was a necessary entity of a wound.

The mortality rate in surgery was so high in England at the time, that if the hospitals in London only had a 26 per cent surgical mortality rate, they expected to be congratulated.

Hospital bulletin boards often carried the message, "The operation was successful, but the patient died from blood poisoning. . . ."

Eventually Lister proved he was right, and he was exonerated and honored. Cambridge and Oxford granted him an LL.D. He was made a Baron and became president of the Royal Society and the British Association for the Advancement of Science. In 1902 he was made an original member of the new Order of Merit. Today, he is honored as the Father of Modern Antiseptic Surgery.

FLORENCE NIGHTINGALE

Florence Nightingale, born of wealthy English parents in 1820, gave up a life of security and luxury to undertake the arduous job of hospital reform.

During England's war with Russia she was sent to the Crimea to be in charge of nursing in an army hospital. Overcoming filth, vermin, overcrowding, and lack of medical and food supplies, Miss Nightingale applied the principles of sanitation and constant care, and within six months brought the hospital death rate from 42 per cent down to 2.2 per cent. Her principles of cleanliness met great resistance from the medical officers.

At night she made the rounds of the wards carrying a lantern, stopping to say a few words to every patient. A soldier wrote, "We lay there by hundreds; but we could kiss her shadow as it fell and lay our heads on the pillow again content." Thus was born the legend of the "Lady with the Lamp."

The sum of $250,000 was raised by England as a tribute to her but she refused to accept the money for herself. Instead, she founded the Florence Nightingale Home for Training Nurses at St. Thomas' Hospital with that money. She also founded a school for nursing in Liverpool.

Florence Nightingale lit a lamp which will burn for all time in the corridors and rooms of hospitals the world over. An heretic who found the hospitals as little better than mortuaries for the poor and destitute, and who left them as institutions of healing.

SISTER ELIZABETH KENNY

Sister Elizabeth Kenny was an Australian nurse and research worker on anterior poliomyelitis. Although she had reasonable success with her therapy in England and Australia, rejection of her therapy by medical physicians brought her to America in 1940. She had hoped that America, young and technologically advanced, would be ready to accept her teaching.

She did not claim a cure for anterior poliomyelitis (infantile paralysis), but until a cure was found, she insisted that her methods provided results after orthodox methods failed. The orthodox method of treatment was splinting the affected extremities, while Sister Kenny's method involved the use of hot packs and muscle education.

Arriving in New York she found that she was unable to get any institution interested in her methods. The National Foundation for Infantile Paralysis could provide money for her work if an accredited institution would request it. No requests came.

She left for Chicago and went to the American Medical Association. The response was almost predictable. The secretary said, "I suppose you're a nun and trying to sell me something. Let me say in advance I'm not buying anything." Sister Kenny replied, "I am not a nun and I have nothing to sell. On the contrary I have something to give, if the people of America will accept it."

Failing to receive any support for her method in Chicago, she went to the Mayo Clinic in Rochester. She was greeted cordially by the head of the orthopedic department, who promptly invited her to address the orthopedists, therapists and other interested physicians. Though her treatment was new to them, they exhibited a sincere interest. Sister Kenny was encouraged.

Visiting polio wards of several St. Paul hospitals, she was allowed to try her treatments on some seemingly hopeless cases. Her results were dramatic. The Minnesota General Hospital, impressed with her results, began using her method of therapy. Finally early in December of 1941 the American Medical Association and the National Foundation for Infantile Paralysis, in a joint radio statement, conceded that Sister Kenny's concept of infantile paralysis was correct. Though she had no university degrees, she was made a faculty member of the University of Minnesota to teach physicians, nurses and technicians her methods of treatment. The American Congress of Physical Therapy awarded her the Distinguished Service Gold Key. Many of her methods of treatment became standard throughout the country.

Her fame was instantaneous. Massive medical assemblies were formed to hear her speak, an institute was named after her, and Hollywood decided to do a movie about her life. Offers poured in from all directions, but she could think only of the crippled bodies which might have been helped if people had listened earlier.

When a reporter asked her what her greatest asset was, she replied with an answer that would gladden the heart of any chiropractor. She replied, "My hands."

In 1952, the United States had one of its worse polio epidemics. About 58,000 children and adults were stricken. The Kenny method, which restored health to thousands of these persons, will live in tribute to a courageous woman who dedicated her life to humanity.

LORRAINE M. GOLDEN

Dr. Lorraine M. Golden, a doctor of chiropractic, might well be considered chiropractic's modern day Florence Nightingale, Madame Curie or Sister Kenny. An intensely compassionate humanitarian, she has dedicated her life to the care of mentally and physically handicapped children, whom she affectionately calls "God's special children."

She acquired an old, unoccupied army hospital site near Louisville, Kentucky, and in 1955 founded Kentuckiana, a private nonprofit, nonsectarian organization which provides free services and care to these children. It provides the widest variety of medical care, including physical therapy, psychological and social counseling of the patients and parents, chiropractic, speech therapy, referral service for medical, dental and surgical attention, optometry, and osteopathy.

The center has cared for over 1,000 children, victims of mental retardation, cerebral palsy, brain injury, asthma, postpolio care, and other illnesses. It also provides regular service to over 275 handicapped children in its clinic, and over 50 children in its special school, which is licensed by the state.

It has always operated in the conviction that "every handicapped child, as a human being regardless of race, social or economic standing, has an innate right to develop to his fullest potential at his own rate of speed."

The services at Kentuckiana are offered without charge. Since 1957, Kentuckiana has provided over $1,100,000 in free services.

A study of Kentuckiana was conducted in May, 1970, by Jerome Smith, assistant professor of the Kent School of Social Work, who praised its "positive and healthy interpersonal relationships." He disproved propaganda that chiropractic claims any "cure-alls" or that it claims any cures for mental retardation. The University of Louisville, through the Kent School, utilizes Kentuckiana as a field placement for its social work students.

One parent decided to take his daughter to the Mayo Clinic for further evaluation after having her at Kentuckiana Center. After an extensive examination at Mayo Clinic, physicians recommended she return to Kentuckiana and continue with the same treatment she had been receiving there. The father returned his daughter to Kentuckiana and became the president of its board of directors.

Dr. Golden has made numerous attempts to obtain financial aid from Crusade for Children, The United Appeal, and the Community Chest, only to be turned down. The Office of Economic Opportunity was enthusiastic about her program until it saw chiropractic care included in Kentuckiana's 18 listed services. Chiropractic is licensed and recognized by law in Kentucky, but that failed to influence the OEO.

Dr. Golden, refusing to go completely medical or chiropractic, has this to say: "No one discipline can make it alone, nor is one discipline superior to another. They must work together."

Kentuckiana is supported entirely by contributions of private individuals and it depends largely on the support of local Mennonites who are willing to work for 50 dollars a month plus room and board.

Dr. Golden's dedication and success with these handicapped children has earned for her the support of local citizens, parents, newspapers, labor unions, civic and religious groups, foundations, corporations, and the chiropractic profession. A group of medical physicians who refer children to her center do so confidentially to avoid the loss of their hospital privileges.

Kentuckiana's greatest obstacle is the economic and political barriers which have been raised against it by organized medicine. Prejudice within healing is a scandalous tragedy, but when it strikes at the hearts of our "little people" it attains a despicability beyond any words that could be used here.

Dr. Joan Partrige, a doctor of chiropractic who is the center's clinical coordinator, said: "If medical science had all the answers, we would not have all these kids here. They'd all be well. None of us has all the answers. When we see changes for the better, sometimes we are dumbfounded. We don't know what happened and neither does anyone else. No one except

God knows what a child is capable of, and no one will ever know if you just put him in an institution."

The majority of the patients at Kentuckiana have been rejected previously by public institutions for financial reasons or as hopeless cases.

Meanwhile our modern day heretical heroine, who says life is too short to quibble over professional prejudices, asks the profoundly moving question, "IF WE DON'T HELP THEM, WHO WILL?" The 1,000 handicapped children who have used Kentuckiana's services might well ask a similar question.

LEO L. SPEARS

Born as a minister's son in the impoverished setting of a log cabin near Tallahassee, Florida, Dr. Spears rose to be one of the great chiropractic pioneers.

Upon graduation from a chiropractic college in 1921, he chose to practice in Denver, Colorado, which was considered the mecca for the sick and suffering. He opened his first office in July of that year, but medical physicians in the building put pressure on the landlord and forced Dr. Spears to move.

Through years of hard work and sacrifice, he prospered to where he had accumulated enough funds to fulfill his greatest dream, the building of a chiropractic hospital.

Then the depression of the 30s struck. The sight of hungry children preyed on Dr. Spears' mind, and as a man who had often known the meaning of hunger, he immediately responded to their needs. He established a bread and milk dispensary for hundreds of needy families with children. The savings he had accumulated through the years eventually was depleted, and with it his immediate plans for construction.

It was another ten years before he was able to build his hospital. Then he was joined by his nephews, Drs. Dan and Howard Spears, who together succeeded in spite of being without the philanthrophic benefits available to other hospitals, a world war which caused building material shortage, and legal maneuvers by organized medicine to try to prevent construction of the building. The hospital was completed in 1943. Soon it was overflowing with patients, and a second building was added in 1949.

Dr. Spears was not the least bit shy about telling others the benefits of chiropractic. At one time, while fighting for the right of veterans to receive chiropractic care, he offered to bring one thousand of his ex-patients to Washington as witnesses. Also, he originated the *Sanigram*, a newspaper which published testimonials of his patients, often those previously declared by medical physicians as "hopeless cases."

The "before and after" testimonials provoked outcries from organized medicine. Medical harassment and legal maneuvers to suppress him failed because the testimonials were factual and thoroughly documented. Though his critics could not explain the reason for his results, they had to concede that he was having apparent success, often after orthodox medicine failed.

His court battles set a significant legal precedence for chiropractic. The Colorado supreme court ruled: "It (chiropractic) may not be arbitrarily limited or discriminated against, and its advocates may lawfully erect and operate buildings and facilities for the treatment, according to its tenets, of patients seeking its aid."

Spears Chiropractic Hospital and clinic, the largest in the world, has treated about 150,000 patients. Yet anyone entering the institution immediately senses an uncommon warmth and dedication to humanity. Service has always been rendered free of charge to sick and crippled children who could not afford this care.

Before Dr. Spears' death on May 16, 1956, he often remarked that his institution must live for hundreds of years. Indeed, the Spears Hospital stands today as majestically as the mountains which graces its background, living in mute testimony to the visions and courage of a healing giant who dared to be an heretic.

CONCLUSION

A world without these giants of the healing arts would certainly be a world which has suffered a great loss for humanity.

Yet, these dedicated people were blindly rejected, persecuted, hated, given insulting nicknames, ridiculed, driven insane, imprisoned, burned at the stake, banished from their country, and had their museums and laboratories destroyed. This was certainly not a fitting reward from a world to which they contributed so much.

The questions might now be asked, "What is the sense of going back 50 or 100 years or more? Why dwell on the unpleasantries of the past? We are in the 1970s; let's live in the present and look to the future!"

We could reply to those questions with more questions. Have we learned anything from all this? Are the tragic lives of these gallant men and women to be in vain? Will we permit history to repeat itself again? Are we to find the 1970s as blind and ignorant as the days of Servetus, Vesalius, Harvey, Bodington, Semmelweis, Nightingale, Kenny and others? How many medical advances have been held back because of blind intolerance, ignorance and violence which discouraged the less determined or courageous? Who can guess?

Dwelling in the past can be meaningless and a waste of time and energy, but if it is done with the specific aim of projecting acquired knowledge into the present and future, then it has significant meaning and purpose. Are we to learn anything that we can project into the present and future regarding chiropractic?

Winston Churchill once observed, "Men occasionally stumble over the truth, but most of them pick themselves up and hurry off as if nothing had happened."

When Alexander Graham Bell introduced the telephone, an evaluation committee of the telegraph company (the ancestor of Western Union) denounced it as "an idiotic, ungainly and impractical device." His ideas were scorned as "extravagant, fanciful predictions, and wild eyed imagination and lack of understanding of the technical and economic fact."

Indeed, man has an incredible record of failure to initially accept the truth. But let us hope, for the sake of humanity, that we all grasp the meaning of the lives presented in this chapter, and take their experiences and project them into the present and future with greater knowledge, understanding, wisdom, and tolerance of investigation. We must all keep our minds open to reason. If we can do this, their lives will indeed have served a noble purpose.

CHAPTER XII

Daniel David Palmer

"In the history of the world, the man who is ahead has always been called an heretic."

ROBERT G. INGERSOLL

IN THE relentless effort of organized medicine to derogate chiropractic, every possible method has been tried, including snide references about the founder of chiropractic. The often-repeated statement goes something like this: "The founder of chiropractic, Dr. Daniel David Palmer, was an uneducated fishpeddler and magnetic healer."

The first reaction expected of the reader is, "How could a profession originating from an uneducated fishmonger and magnetic healer be any good?" This is precisely the reaction organized medicine encourages when it propagates that statement so frequently. Now let's examine the facts.

SELF EDUCATED

It must be remembered that Dr. Palmer lived in the 1800s when a formal education was the exception, not the rule. All the medical doctors in the 1800s would be considered inadequate and incompetent quacks by today's standards. Remember, of the 155 medical schools of 1910 all but 31 were considered diploma mills, and standards then were far from what they are today.

Some of the greatest geniuses had no formal education, but through self education attained great accomplishments in life. Dr. Palmer was such a man. He read a wide variety of books on healing, becoming remarkably well oriented.

One of America's most renowned presidents, Abraham Lincoln, had less than one year of formal education and was a farmer and rail splitter. President Harry Truman was a haberdasher and never attended college. Are we to derogate them because of this?

If we searched the world over could we find a more revered and dedicated nurse than Florence Nightingale, the mother of nursing? Her total nurse's training consisted of only 3½ months! By modern standards she would be declared totally incompetent, yet in her day she was the head of a hospital for invalid gentlemen in London, later in charge of 38 nurses at an army hospital. She was the founder of two nursing schools and helped establish many training centers. She wrote extensively, was responsible for obtaining badly needed hospital reforms, received the British Order of Merit and was granted the freedom of the city of London. Are we to deny her great service to humanity because she did not meet the standards of the 1970s? Of course not. Nor is it logical to do the same with the founder of chiropractic based on the educational standards of another era. Miss Nightingale lived in the same era as Dr. Palmer. She died in 1910, just three years before his death.

Thomas A. Edison never progressed beyond the second grade in school, yet he became the greatest inventive genius of all time. He acquired 1,097 patents and we are using all but four of these today. Are we to deny such genius?

Anton V. Leeuwenhoek had no formal education. He was a shopkeeper and salesman and an exciseman who measured wine casks. But he developed the microscope and carried on monumental research in bacteriology, and later became known as "The Father of Microscopy." Few men of great formal education have contributed more than he did to the world of healing. Are we to deny his contributions?

Unfortunately, the medical textbooks of Dr. Daniel Palmer's era had many errors and the existing drugs were mostly worthless or even dangerous. Physicians with the most sophisticated formal education of that day subscribed to some of the most erroneous medical theories. We need only to reflect upon the lives of Semmelweis, Pasteur, Nightingale and Lister who were ridiculed for speaking the truth. Dr. Daniel Palmer was a young man of 20 when Semmelweis died in a mental hospital trying to expose ignorance. Louis Pasteur died in 1895, the year chiropractic was founded. Also the same year chiropractic was founded, Dr. Wilhelm Roentgen, a German scientist, discovered the x-ray, only to be criticized publicly for invading the privacy of the boudoir with invisible rays. The laryngoscope, a valuable diagnostic instrument, was ridiculed as a "worthless toy."

Such was the era of Dr. Daniel David Palmer. Realizing many of the errors and shortcomings of the medical teachings of his time, he wrote about them in his book, *The Science, Art and Philosophy of Chiropractic.*

THE GROCER

Dr. Palmer's early years were spent working as a grocer. He frequently delivered groceries which included fish, so you might say he qualified to be called a "fish peddler."

In regard to the early occupations of professional men, the first surgeons were bloodletters and barbers. The early surgeons applied leeches to the patient's body as one of their methods of treatment. Many of the early physicians were itinerant health peddlers of low repute, selling their services from door to door.

THE MAGNETIC HEALER

The age in which Dr. Palmer lived was governed by unbelievable ignorance and false information on healing.

Separating fact from fiction in the writings of that age often was difficult. What we now view as obvious truths were not so obvious years ago.

Magnetic healing was very much the vogue of the day and Dr. Palmer had considerable success with many people, though he was not satisfied with it and was constantly searching for a better way.

Today, magnetic healing is recognized by many authorities as the first step toward the psychoanalytical and psychological methods of healing.

CONCLUSION

Dr. Daniel David Palmer was a brilliant, self-educated man whose genius and penetrating mind set forth a basic principle in healing which stands stronger today than ever before. The inferences to his humble beginning, in an effort to derogate him and chiropractic, reflect adversely on the good taste and integrity of those who have sought to demolish his reputation and do away with chiropractic.

Where else but in the distorted minds of propagandists could such innocent information be prostituted into an attempt at derogation of a worthy profession? Only warped minds would try to attack the fine profession of surgery by saying its founders were bloodletters and leech carriers, or try to discredit nursing by reference to the fact that Florence Nightingale died with neurosyphilis. Shall we downgrade Abraham Lincoln because of his humble beginning? Shall we try to downgrade medical doctors by saying the first medical physicians were often illiterate, door-to-door health peddlers who were held in low esteem?

It would be vicious and unfair to attack noble persons or professions in this manner, yet this is precisely the tactic used by the propagandists in their attacks on chiropractic. In doing so, they have stooped to the lowest imaginable form of gutter journalism.

CHAPTER XIII

Medical Plagiarism, Monopoly and Bigotry

CHIROPRACTIC

SKEPTICS of chiropractic have asked, "If chiropractic is as good as all that, why didn't medicine adopt it years ago?"

The answer is simple. It is a historical fact that physicians have never been quick to adopt many truths, in spite of overwhelming proof which was presented at the time. We need only refer to the chapter on "Heretical Giants" as evidence of this fact.

It is a fact, however, that the medical profession is beginning to adopt many of the teachings of chiropractic. In 1968, a group of prominent medical physicians formed the North American Academy of Manual Medicine which is devoted to study, teach, research and advance spinal manipulative procedures within medicine.

More striking proof of this was the formation and meeting of the First Congress of the International Federation of Manual Medicine in 1968. The congress, held in London, England, was attended by hundreds of enthusiastic medical physicians from all parts of the world. Its purpose was to advance spinal manipulation within medicine, under a name other than chiropractic or osteopathy.

An increasing number of medical physicians are using spinal manipulative procedures or "adjustments" under the banner of physiatry, manipulative medicine, physical medicine, manual medicine, orthopedic manipulation, rachiotherapy, vertebrotherapy, etc. Whatever you may wish to call it, it still represents basic spinal manipulative or adjustive procedures that chiropractors have been successfully using for over 75 years.

Seminars and symposia on spinal manipulation have been given for medical doctors. The Iowa Medical School in October, 1970, taught "The Art and Technique of Spinal Manipulation." The San Francisco Medical Center gave a seminar in 1965 entitled "Joint Manipulation and Prospective."

A symposium on spinal manipulation for medical doctors was held at St. Mary's Hospital and Medical Center in San Francisco on March 16–17, 1971. It was entitled "Common Pain Syndromes and Joint Manipulation." It is especially noteworthy that this symposium was endorsed by the AMA.

A prominent chiropractic spokesman, Dr. Leonard Savage, addressed a University of California symposium on March 27, 1971. The symposium was attended by faculty members and students of the University of California medical, dental, nursing, pharmacy and social welfare schools.

Dr. Savage noted that the AMA had endorsed a symposium on spinal manipulation held just 10 days earlier and went on to charge that such action represented "an incredible demonstration of duplicity, deceit and deliberate dishonesty." He said, "When the AMA continues to attack our profession, one which spends four years teaching the principles and techniques of manipulation including full diagnostic training, and then endorses a medical presentation of 3½ hours on the same course of treatment, its self-serving hypocrisy is revealed." He went on to say, "The advertising of the symposium is misleading in causing medical doctors to believe they may be qualified to perform spinal manipulations after a few hours attendance at a series of superficial lectures and demonstrations." He explained that such seminars were "irresponsible and potentially dangerous" and if they thought their malpractice premiums were high then, they had better have second thoughts before applying crude manipulative skills to live patients. He explained that if they presented their seminar in depth for some four academic years it would have value, but then it would become a course in chiropractic.

Finally, Dr. Savage suggested the best way the medical experts could make their brief symposia valuable would be to conclude the programs by saying, "Now that you have seen the significance of joint manipulation, we urge you to contact a competent chiropractic doctor in your neighborhood and refer to him those patients who would benefit from his methods."

Prominent medical journals and recognized textbooks of medical learning throughout the world are also referring to spinal manipulative procedures in the care of human ailments.

Chiropractic has been legally licensed and regulated as a separate and distinct science for many years. It is also common knowledge that medicine has rejected the spinal manipulative approach to healing as not being a part of medicine. How can medicine legally infringe upon another profession's method of healing by adopting spinal manipulative methods, the very methods they have for so long emphatically rejected and renounced, ridiculed and even condemned? The answer to that question lies in the often vague or liberal interpretation of the state laws for medicine which were written in the 1800s. The state of Washington, however, has a law prohibiting medical physicians from practicing chiropractic.

Thorp McClusky, in his book *Your Health and Chiropractic*, noted that chiropractic can well be summarized in the words of Charles F. Kettering, President of General Motors Research Corporation, when he once said, "First they tell you that you are wrong—and they can prove it. Then they tell you that you are right—but it's not important. Then they tell you it is important—but they've known it all these years."

PODIATRY (formerly chiropody)

The early medical physicians believed it beneath their dignity to treat foot conditions. They rejected foot care as not within the realm of medicine. Thus, chiropody (now known as podiatry) was born out of ignorance and rejection by early medical physicians.

As foot care came into vogue, the podiatrist not only found the medical doctors treating foot conditions, but also borrowing many of his surgical techniques.

Today, the podiatrist finds himself with privileges and staff membership in some hospitals while in other medical hospitals he must be cosponsored by a medical doctor who will oversee his surgery, a surgery which often was developed by podiatrists.

The standard curriculum of a podiatry college is of high caliber and similar to that of a medical school, but with emphasis on the feet, and on general body maladies which may stem from ailments of the feet. In spite of this, many physicians question the necessity of the podiatrist beyond the care of corns, calluses and toe nails, and seek to handle the more glamorous foot conditions such as spurs and tenomyotomys.

The March 18, 1971, *New England Journal of Medicine* carried an article which discussed podiatry. Although objective and generally favorable to podiatry, it still asked, "Why does podiatry exist at all? Would physicians provide the needed foot care? Could technicians working under a physician's supervision do part of this work? Could the orthopedist take care of all the bunions and hammer toes?"

Thus, while podiatry is gaining recognition and staff membership in many medical hospitals and there appears to be a close cooperation between these two professions, certain undercurrents smack of medical plagiarism and monopoly.

OPTOMETRY

In 1955, the American Medical Association in convention passed some resolutions against the profession of optometry. These resolutions declared a virtual boycott of the optometric profession. They forbade medical doctors from teaching in optometric colleges, writing in optometric journals, and lecturing before optometric societies.

Here is the exact wording of Resolution 77, adopted by the AMA House of Delegates in June, 1955: "RESOLVED, that it is unethical for any doctor of medicine to teach in any school or college of optometry, or to lecture in any optometric organization, or to contribute scientific material to the optometric literature, or in any way to impart technical medical knowledge to nonmedical practitioners."

Coronet Magazine carried an article entitled, "The Battle for Your Eyes." This article illustrated the affect the resolutions had upon the optometrists and the people they served. One optometrist who was with a research company in Linden, N.J. for 13 years was fired because he could not "associate" with the medical men on the staff.

The Lions Clubs throughout the country were sponsoring a glaucoma screening project but the ophthalmologists flatly stated that if the optometrists participated in this program, they would not.

Meanwhile the ophthalmologists, through the National Medical Foundation for Eye Care, were undermining public trust in optometry by insisting that only the medical doctor is qualified to diagnose the absence or presence of glaucoma and that drops were necessary for a more "complete" and "accurate" eye refraction. Since optometrists cannot use drugs or "drops" in all the states, it was implied that only the medical doctors could properly examine eyes.

People were led to believe that the eye drops which the ophthalmologists were using in examinations were beneficial, yet harmless. It is an established fact that eye drops are mydriatics and mydriatics can initiate acute glaucoma.

Meanwhile, the offices of the ophthalmologists were flooded with more patients than they could accommodate, and they realized they needed assistance. They could not hire optometrists because their own resolution prohibited them from doing so. So what could they do?

Their problem was directed to the judicial council of the AMA, which reported on December 19, 1960, that "It is unethical for a doctor to hire an optometrist as an assistant, if the optometrist is held out to the public or the doctor's patient as a doctor of optometry or a licensed optometrist. It is not unethical, however, for a doctor of medicine to hire one who may have been trained or who may have a degree in optometry if the individual so hired is not held out or does not hold himself out to the public as an optometrist." And so they added insult to injury by saying the ophthalmologists could hire optometrists to work for them provided their true identity as optometrists was in no way revealed to the patient.

On July 24, 1964, a $90 million lawsuit was brought against the AMA and eight Chicago ophthalmologists charging them with violation of the Sherman Antitrust Act. This was instituted by a group of optometrists with the principal plaintiff being Dr. Cyrus Bass of Chicago.

Before filing the lawsuit, the plaintiff asked two patients to cooperate in an experiment. He wanted to see how deeply rooted was the discrimination against optometry. He wanted to see whether the ophthalmologists would behave ethically if they thought optometrists were involved.

His experiment called for the patients to go to an ophthalmologist, get their eyes examined, and obtain the prescribed glasses. Then they would go with these new glasses to a second ophthalmologist, have their eyes examined again, and obtain the glasses he prescribed. Of course, the patient would tell each ophthalmologist that his glasses had just recently been prescribed by an "optometrist."

The first patient visited six ophthalmologists and five prescribed glasses. The second patient, a diabetic, visited six ophthalmologists and also received five pairs of glasses. The diabetic patient told these ophthalmologists that he was suffering dizzy spells, but only one of them indicated it might be caused by the diabetic condition and recommended he see his physician. In addition to the new glasses, five ophthalmologists offered unsolicited derogatory remarks about optometry in general. Two of the ophthalmologists were visited by both patients, thus bringing to eight the number of ophthalmologists prescribing glasses. Eight ophthalmologists were either unable to agree on the diagnosis of a simple eye refraction or were practicing fraud. These eight along with the AMA, were named defendants in this lawsuit.

Two vital court decisions were decided in favor of the optometrists. The AMA realized that this group of optometrists was creating a serious threat to them. Meanwhile, the American Optometric Association was engaged in efforts to eliminate the prejudice against optometry.

Finally, the AMA House of Delegates in June, 1966, introduced Resolution 107 which dissolved the previous resolutions against optometrists. Then in November, 1966, the AMA Judicial Council issued two rulings. The first was that ophthalmologists may employ an optometrist provided the optometrist holds himself out as an optometrist and not as a medical doctor. The second was that medical physicians may now teach in recognized schools of optometry.

In 1967, with the boycott against optometry removed, the law suit against the AMA was terminated.

Does it sound too incredible to be true? You may check for yourself by reading *Cyrus Bass et al. v. American Medical Association,* 64C1279, United States District Court, Northern District of Illinois, Eastern Division. It is a matter of public record.

Although optometry has been successful in improving its interprofessional relationship with organized medicine, it must still maintain constant vigil for its rights and the rights of patients. The August 9, 1971, issue of the *American Medical News* (an AMA publication) clearly illustrated this point when it revealed that a group of Houston, Texas, optometrists had filed a $3 million antitrust suit against the Houston Ophthalmological Society.

OSTEOPATHY

Organized medicine's position concerning the osteopathic profession has changed from open attack to the current subtle tactics of absorption and elimination.

During the open attack phase in trying to eliminate osteopathy the official position of the AMA was that all osteopathic colleges were inadequate and that all osteopathic physicians were cultists, and that medical doctors could not associate with or teach in schools of osteopathy.

As osteopathy grew in numbers, sophistication and general acceptance, the AMA realized that its hostile approach had not been successful. It then reverted to the more subtle "kill with kindness" approach.

The judicial council of the AMA reported that the best way to eliminate osteopathy was to have medical physicians teach in its schools. Dr. Frank A. MacDonald of California proposed taking over the College of Osteopathic Physicians and Surgeons in Los Angeles and granting M.D. degrees to the 2,400 osteopaths in that state. With uninhibited frankness and boldness he explained that this approach could eliminate all of the osteopathic colleges, and if it were successful in California it could be done elsewhere. After all, amalgamation had already worked, earlier in this century, with the homeopaths. Once they were absorbed into the medical (allopathic) profession they quietly disappeared as an alternate school of practice.

How could the AMA create a merger if its own policies specifically prohibited its state societies from associating with osteopaths? The solution was simple. In 1961 the AMA House of Delegates abruptly reversed its official position on osteopathy saying not all osteopaths were cultists after all, only those who did not practice "scientific medicine." Without defining its interpretation of "scientific medicine," the AMA House of Delegates went on to declare that not all osteopathic colleges were inadequate after all.

Suddenly one college, the College of Osteopathic Physicians and Surgeons in Los Angeles, became so adequate that it was immediately converted into a medical school and empowered to confer M.D. degrees for $65.00 apiece on some 2,000 California osteopaths who chose to enter the allopathic profession. As part of the deal the osteopathic board of examiners discontinued the licensing of new osteopaths. With the passing or retirement of the remaining osteopaths who chose not to go into the allopathic profession, osteopathy's future existence in that state was severely threatened.

This, of course, whetted organized medicine's appetite. In the state of Washington a similar merger plan went into effect. Fifty-four osteopaths were influenced to break away from the existing Washington Osteopathic Medical Association, form their own group and then merge with the Washington State Medical Society. They formed the Washington College of Physicians and Surgeons which had no regular faculty, no established curriculum and no permanent facilities. Then these osteopaths could take a "postgraduate" course at this "paper college" for 12 Saturday afternoons and be granted an M.D. degree. Meanwhile, the Washington Medical Board of Examiners recognized this paper college.

The osteopathic profession, realizing the mergers and "paper colleges" were part of a plan to take over osteopathy by the medical profession, instituted legal action to preserve its own identity. Ironically, it also was preserving the integrity of the M.D. degree as well.

The legal action taken by the osteopathic profession had significant effect. On November 8, 1967, the Supreme Court of the state of New York ruled against recognition of the $65.00 M.D. diploma from California. Up to this time, the New York department of education was the only state that ever gave this spurious diploma any kind of recognition.

Shortly thereafter, the Washington Supreme Court overruled the state's board of medical examiners which had previously recognized the paper college.

Finally, the California osteopaths who chose not to go into the allopathic profession brought suit against the California Medical Association. A California district court decision in 1971 stated that the state acting on behalf of the medical examiners failed to show why new osteopaths could not be licensed in California. Licensing was resumed in 1974 breaking medicine's monopolistic attempts on osteopathy.

In July, 1969, the American Osteopathic Association House of Delegates adopted a resolution warning that any American Osteopathic Association member accepting membership of any kind in the American Medical Association or its affiliates would be acting against the interest of the AOA and would be subject to discipline, which might even be expulsion.

In May, 1965, March, 1968, and August, 1970, the American Osteopathic Association released its official statements of AOA-AMA past and present relationships in the form of a "white paper."

The last paragraph of the most recent "white paper" summarized the position of the osteopaths eloquently when it said, "Actually, the AMA's policies, past and present, could be compared to the difference between the Neanderthal man who slew his rivals with a club and the infinitely more sophisticated Borgias who dispatched their enemies by inviting them to a good dinner heavily laced with poison. The lyrics may have changed, but the melody remains the same."

CONCLUSION

How much better it would be for humanity if optometry, podiatry, osteopathy and chiropractic simply could exert their full energies to advancing their professions, rather than fight the suppressive and monopolistic attempts of organized medicine. What a tragic waste of time, energy and money, especially during a national health crisis.

Regardless of the reluctance of organized medicine to recognize and admit it, the fact is that health and illness are the collective responsibility of the medical doctor, the doctor of chiropractic, the doctor of osteopathy, the doctor of dentistry, the doctor of podiatry, the doctor of optometry, the nurse, the medical and dental technicians, the pharmacist, the dietitian, and of those in other health-allied professions. It is no longer the private domain of the doctor of medicine.

Congressman David King of Utah asked the question, "Is there any reason why the same freedom should not exist in the field of health as exists in business or politics, or religion, or anything else? Is there any reason why one single approach to the problem of health, backed by powerful financial interests, should be given a complete monopoly?".

Dr. Benjamin Rush, a medical physician and one of the signers of the Declaration of Independence, once said: "To restrict the art of healing to one class of men and deny equal privilege to others constitute the bastille of medical science. Such restrictions are fragments of monarchy and have no place in a republic."

CHAPTER XIV

Health Abuse

UNITED NATIONS POPULATION AND VITAL STATISTICS

THE United Nations publishes a *Population and Vital Statistics Report* available at book stores or through the United Nations in New York. The price is $1.

The July 1, 1970, edition provides some revealing and shocking statistics which should be of interest to everyone.

Thirty-five out of 36 North American countries reported their death rates with the United Nations. The lone exception was Haiti.

The registered death rate in the United States was 9.5 deaths per 1,000. Only three countries in North America had a higher registered death rate than the United States, in spite of the fact that the United States enjoys the lowest registered infant mortality rate of all these countries. (The United States and Canada's infant mortality rate is 20.8.)

The United Nations figures are shown on the next page.

The conclusion is inevitable that while we have been able to save our newly born children through modern obstetrical procedures, our adults are dying faster than in almost every other country in North America. This is a sad commentary on the wealthiest and most medically sophisticated country of them all.

Country	*Registered Death Rate (per 1,000)*	*Infant Mortality Rate (per 1,000)*
Antigua	8.4	45.4
Bahamas	5.8	45.8
Barbados	8.1	45.6
Bermuda	8.0	23.6
British Honduras	6.1	51.8
British Virgin Islands	8.8	66.7
Canada	7.3	20.8
Cayman Islands	4.0	(not given)
Costa Rica	7.1	62.3
Cuba	6.4	37.6
Dominica	8.2	44.7
Dominican Republic	6.9	72.6
El Salvador	9.9	59.2
Greenland	8.1	70.1
Grenada	8.0	34.1
Guadeloupe	8.1	49.6
Guatemala	13.3	89.0
Haiti	(no registered rates submitted)	
Honduras	8.4	35.5
Jamaica	7.7	32.5
Martinique	7.2	37.1
Mexico	9.1	65.7
Montserrat	9.4	37.9
Netherlands Antilles	5.0	22.2
Nicaragua	8.0	55.4
Panama	7.3	40.8
Canal Zone	2.3	(not given)
Puerto Rico	5.6	28.3
St. Kitts-Nevis-Anguilla	7.9	59.3
St. Lucia	7.1	42.4
St. Pierre and Miquelon	10.1	(not given)
St. Vincent	9.3	73.7
Trinidad and Tobago	6.8	35.8
Turks and Caicos Islands	6.8	(not given)
United States of America	9.5	20.8
U.S. Virgin Islands	7.9	27.7

The United Nations' World Health Organization's figures also shows that the United States longevity rate is steadily declining in rank among the nations of the world. The male life expectancy was 13th in the world in 1963. In 1964 it dropped to 18th. In 1965 it dropped to 21st. In 1971 it dropped to 22nd!

Statistics compiled by the United States Department of Health, Education and Welfare indicate that life expectancy for a man of 65 has been decreasing since 1952.

Our diminishing health is not confined to the elderly. Dr. Julius Richmond, Dean of the State University of New York Upstate Medical Center College of Medicine, compiled the following data on children in the United States: Half of them under the age of 15 have never visited a dentist, eleven million children between the ages of 15 and 17 have eye disorders requiring medical attention, two million have untreated hearing defects, nearly three million have untreated speech disorders, 4.6 million have untreated emotional disturbances, and two million have untreated orthopedic problems.

President Eisenhower's Advisory Committee on Youth Fitness conducted physical fitness tests on 7,000 children in the United States, Italy, Austria and Switzerland, and found that 6 out of 10 American children failed the fitness test, compared to less than 1 out of 10 in the other countries. The July, 1956, *Reader's Digest*, commenting on this physical fitness test, quoted President Eisenhower as being "shocked" by these figures.

Analysts "prove" and "disprove" different theories concerning these statistics, but one fact that cannot be dismissed is that with all our wealth and medical sophistication, we in America are not as healthy as we should be.

NUTRITION ABUSE

We are grossly negligent in our eating habits. We not only overeat but often our diet is not properly balanced with nutritious food.

Dr. Roger J. Williams, a University of Texas nutrition expert, spoke before the National Academy of Science saying he fed 64 rats exclusively on our commercial "enriched" bread. He revealed that within 90 days, 40 of the rodents died and the survivors were severely stunted. Our "staff of life" cannot even support rats!

In a control experiment, 64 other rats were fed exclusively on bread with small amounts of vitamins, minerals and amino acids added. All but three were alive and thriving at the end of 90 days. Dr. Williams said that bakers could supplement their bread with the nutrients he used for about three cents a loaf. Dr. Williams said the Food and Drug Administration (FDA) and the medical profession encourage an atmosphere in which the importance of proper nutrition is ignored in spite of modern research proving its necessity.

Now, let's follow the routine day of many typical Americans. Perhaps you might even see yourself here. For breakfast we have coffee, a sweet roll and a cigarette and rush off to work. For lunch, we have a sandwich made of the so-called "enriched" bread, soft drink or coffee. Of course, we must have our morning and afternoon coffee breaks with more coffee, more cigarettes and more sweet rolls. We are convinced that without such treats we could not finish the day. The evening meal generally includes plenty of starchy potatoes, fried meats, bread, butter and dessert. Such meals are perfect for packing extra weight on our bodies. Wholesome, vitamin rich foods often are neglected.

We bleach our flour, polish our rice, refine our sugar, peel our carrots and potatoes and by so doing remove many of the vital nutrients from these foods. Those criticizing such common practices are labeled as some sort of health faddists.

The Medical College of Wisconsin, in Milwaukee, in cooperation with TOPS, Inc. conducted the largest study of obesity ever taken. (TOPS is a weight watchers organization; the initials stand for Take Off Pounds Sensibly.) Dr. Alfred A. Rimm, head of the researchers, found that over 60 million

Americans are overweight, and 25 million of these are more than 15 per cent over their best weight. Dr. Rimm said, "Since it has been demonstrated that obesity is associated with increased morbidity and mortality, it is clearly a disease; in this country, it is of epidemic proportion." He added that obesity is probably more critical to national health than undernutrition.

Have you ever tried to take out a life insurance policy while 50 pounds overweight? Insurance companies make it their business to know what the chances are of your dying, and their computers tell them to avoid you because you are a bad risk. If you are between the ages of 45 and 50 and 10 pounds overweight, your death rate is 8 per cent higher. If you are 20 pounds overweight, it is 18 per cent higher. If you are 30 pounds overweight, it is 28 per cent higher. If you are 50 pounds overweight, it is 56 per cent higher!

This is it. We promise to lose 50 pounds. Should we go on a diet? Nonsense, we are convinced that it is our "glands." We come from a family of heavies and the only way to reduce is to use weight reducing pills. We go to our family doctor who so obligingly sees that we are furnished with a nice supply of pills. We are convinced that now we can continue to eat what we want, even making occasional gluttons of ourselves, and lose weight.

MEDICATION ABUSE

George P. Larrick, former commissioner of the United States Food and Drug Administration, said: "I know it is common to speak of the 'good old days' of snake oil and soothing syrup as though they were gone forever. . . . The amazing fact is that to a very great extent those 'good old days' are still with us."

Early drug advertising was unregulated and frequently fraudulent, limited only by the creative imagination of the patent-medicine promoter. More recently, strides have been made to protect the consumer against definitely harmful drugs. Yet, almost no protection exists against ineffective drugs, and very little protection exists against deceptive and misleading drug advertising. This includes ethical drugs, those advertised only to medical physicians and pharmacists.

The ineffectiveness of the FD&C Law (Food, Drug & Cosmetics) is illustrated by a conversation at a pharmacists production manager's meeting: "I tell you, we don't have anything to worry about. To this day, that section of the law is not well defined. You can stand there and piss in the batch and turn around and shake the FDA inspector's hand. He's going to tell you that's not right, but when you go to court, they won't find you guilty . . . They have not been able to make this law stick!"

Joseph Addison, English essayist, poet and dramatist of the early eighteenth century, wrote of the patent-medicine promoters: "Had all these advertisers arrived to that skill they pretend to, they would have no need for so many years successively to publish to the world the place of their abode and the virtues of their medicines." Indeed, patent-medicine advertising today has expanded to a multimillion dollar a year business.

The persistent advertising of drugs has been successful, at least to the drug peddlers. We have been conditioned to accept drugs as a contemporary panacea. When our bodies begin to show signs or symptoms of distressed function we tend to concern ourselves with the symptoms and how to suppress them with drugs, rather than even question their possible cause and prevention. Chiropractic health care which stresses cause and prevention of body ailments is too often ignored or forgotten, and even condemned. If we suffer from heartburn, nervous stomach, and indigestion which may be associated with our rapid pace, nervous tension, and improper diet, we fail to concern ourselves with the cause, and instead turn to alkalizers and tranquilizers. If we have a headache which could be from a multitude of causes, we take an aspirin. If we go to bed and can't sleep, we "pop" a sleeping pill. In the morning if we can't seem to stay awake we take a wake-up pill, and during the day we have pills to stimulate or relax us depending on the need. If we are constipated, we take a laxative instead of seeking out and eliminating the cause. If we suffer from body aches and pains, which may be nature's distress signal, we take a pain killer or muscle relaxant. If we have a low grade fever, which is one of nature's way of fighting an infection, we take an aspirin to bring the temperature down. Finally, if we get run down and our body is taken over by physical or emotional exhaustion, viruses, bacteria or whatever, we take the appropriate antibiotic, sulfa drug, stimulant or symptom suppressor to "feel better."

President Nixon, who receives regular spinal manipulative care from an osteopath, told Congress, "We should build a true 'health' system, not a 'sickness' system alone. We should work to maintain health and not merely to restore it." Yet, modern society too often feels that proper rest, exercise, fresh air, proper diet, a minimum use of drugs, chiropractic care, and more faith in our natural recuperative powers was all right for Hippocrates and grandma. "But this is the 1970s," we seem to say, "and the drug industry with its pills has, for us, a solution to every problem."

Finally, we find ourselves part of a drug oriented society that seems to have a magic pill for everything. It is a society with more than 22,000 drug products on the market. It is a society in which each family has 29 different kinds of pills in their medicine cabinet, and according to *Newsweek* magazine of September 8, 1969, is subsidizing an annual $5 billion prescription drug industry. It is a society that averages four prescriptions a year for every man, woman and child in America. And the latter statistics do not include drugs received in hospitals. It is a society that annually consumes approximately TWO MILLION POUNDS OF MOOD DRUGS to stimulate or sedate our body functions. It is a society in which physicians write prescriptions for 13 billion barbiturates and amphetamines each year, enough to keep every adult and child in this country under the influence of these medications for over one month. It is a society that consumes an incredible TEN MILLION POUNDS OF ASPIRIN ANNUALLY, or in other words, FIVE THOUSAND TONS OF ASPIRIN! Do you realize how large a pile a ton of coal amounts to? We live in a society in which 5,000 such piles of aspirin and 1,000 piles of amphetamines and barbiturates are consumed annually. Tragically, it is also a society of iatrogenic diseases, drug addiction and a steadily declining life expectancy among the nations of the world.

DEEP CONCERN

Many of the most outstanding, knowledgeable and distinguished members of the healing world have registered alarm in this current trend. Here are a few of their comments:

Dr. Herbert Ratner, professor of preventive medicine at the Stritch School of Medicine said, "The United States is the worst place in the world to have a nonserious disease . . . It is generally recognized that America is the most overmedicated, overoperated and most overinoculated country in the world." He also added that while we are the wealthiest nation in the world, we are also one of the unhealthiest.

Hobart A. Reimann, M.D., of the Hahnemann Medical College in Philadelphia said 90 per cent of antibiotics are given unnecessarily.

Dr. William Boyd, one of America's most renowned and internationally famous pathologists and author of *A Textbook of Pathology, an Introduction to Medicine*, criticized the regard for antibiotics as cure-alls. He said that allergies to drugs are increasing to the point that they are said to exceed bacterial disease in number, and that if we continue to fool with nature, we must pay the penalty. In reference to medications he added, "What is powerful for good can be potent for evil."

Dr. Robert H. Moser, professor of internal medicine from

Baylor University in Texas and prominent author of *Diseases of Medical Progress*, reflected the same concern. He spoke of unfavorable side-effects of drugs, sometimes even fatal, and of the frequent indiscriminate use of drugs by physicians without regard to their dangerous potential. He also attacked the use of antibiotics for trivial upper respiratory infections and other minor ailments.

The use of high powered drugs for minor infections can be compared to killing a fly on your piano with a heavy club instead of a fly swatter. Either way kills the fly, but what about the piano?

Dr. David M. Spain is the author of *The Complications of Modern Medical Practice*. The renowned pathologist and author said that iatrogenic diseases (medication-caused disease) are on par with bacterial disease as cause of human ailments and that 50 out of 1,000 beds in hospitals are occupied by people with medication-caused illness.

Dr. James Roth, M.D., professor of gastroenterology at the University of Pennsylvania School of Medicine, said that all people who take aspirin in almost any form will bleed internally in small amounts. Experimentation on cats showed 84 per cent had erosion of stomach lining and superficial ulcers, and that buffering agents did not help.

Dr. René Menguy, professor of surgery at the University of Chicago, conducted 10 years of research into the effects of aspirin. He concluded that while even the occasional aspirin user can suffer blood loss, the person who takes one or two aspirin a day may lose four to five teaspoons of blood every week. Although most people can lose this amount without ill effects, some will react severely, he said. According to a survey at the University of Chicago, one out of every seven persons who come to a hospital emergency room with severe stomach or intestinal bleeding, has a bleeding problem caused by the use of aspirin. Dr. Menguy estimated that at least 1,000 ulcer patients died annually from these complications.

Dr. Vernon M. Smith, professor of medicine at the University of Maryland, said aspirin may prove to be one cause of heart attacks, strokes, and excessive or irregular menstrual bleeding.

In another study, Dr. J. Lawrence Naiman of the Temple University School of Medicine reported that stomach bleeding in children by recent ingestion of aspirin can restrict proper blood platelet functioning and prolong bleeding time.

Dr. Paul Stolley of Johns Hopkins Medical School said that 95 per cent of those who consult a medical physician for a common cold are given prescriptions, and 90 per cent of those drugs prescribed are antibiotics and antihistamines, which have been found through controlled tests to be ineffective or the possible cause of side effects.

Dr. Dale Consol, medical director of Squibb Laboratories, said, "Doctors and the public are subjected to a constant barrage of new drugs, some worthless and others with greater potential for harm than good."

The book entitled, *The Therapeutic Nightmare* by Morton Mintz, criticized the "irrational and massive use of prescription drugs that may be worthless, injurious, or even lethal" and the AMA for its lack of initiative in assessing the value of new drugs.

Dr. Charles May, prominent pediatrician and former editor of *Pediatrics*, said one of the pharmaceutical industry's "tricks of the trade" is to quote inferior research articles in medical literature to support claims "even when superior work is available to refute them."

In November, 1971, Senator Gaylord Nelson of Wisconsin addressed the Senate: "There is an inevitable tendency, no matter how conscientious the firm, to emphasize the positive features and deemphasize the negative. . . . Many of the people they engage to do their testing are equally anxious to secure additional contracts for drug testing. . . . A physician who turns in unfavorable reports on the drugs he is testing may not have his contract renewed . . . In case after case, some firms have been guilty of misrepresenting, distorting, and even withholding information developed in their testing of drugs, which might in any way retard or prevent an approval to market. Injury and death have resulted from such action."

Vice President Hubert Humphrey, himself a pharmacist, said in 1962:

"The more we have examined the handling of new drugs by the Food and Drug Administration, the more we have been surprised, shocked and disappointed . . . Often, testing has been going on in a manner which should have sent shivers down the spine of the medical profession. . . .

"Drugs intended for use by victims of chronic disease—day after day, year after year—were released by FDA even before—I repeat, before chronic toxicity tests had been completed on animals. . . . shocking reports of injuries to test patients, as received by drug companies, have often gone unreported to the FDA, or have been downgraded by skillfully contrived half-truths, or have been reported accurately to FDA, but virtually ignored.

"Drugs have been approved which the FDA now admits should never have been approved. Drugs have been kept on the market after FDA admits they should have been eliminated."

Dr. Albert H. Holland, former FDA medical director said: "The naive belief that if the product was not good the FDA would prohibit its sales is just not realistic. FDA labors long and diligently to protect the public, but the fact of the matter is, it is completely impossible for FDA to check every batch of every product of every manufacturer that is marketed."

The criticism of worthless or dangerous drugs on the market was dramatically called to public attention in November, 1970, when the Food and Drug Administration, Bureau of Drugs, condemned 369 drugs and ordered them off the market. The FDA commissioned a research study by the National Academy of Sciences, which formed a National Research Council Drug Efficacy Study Group. Dr. Robert K. Cannan, administrative head of that study, found that mislabeling generally involved misleading and devious advertising on drugs. The *Chicago Today* newspaper on November 29, 1970, quoted Dr. Cannan as saying, "Many of the claims made for these drugs are indefensible and some of the advertisements turned my stomach."

This is a significant fact. Drug manufacturers spend nearly $800 million a year promoting their drugs in medical journals. While it is true that many medical doctors take postgraduate work to keep up with the latest medical developments, the Fond du Lac Study of Wisconsin showed that most doctors received most of their information on drugs from this drug advertisement literature. Therefore, the patient is too often treated by the well-meaning medical doctor who prescribes medicines on the basis of abusive advertisements which are intended to "sell" the physician rather than educate him.

To complicate this already serious situation, Dr. Dale G. Friend of Harvard Medical School stated, "From the eight-thousand drugs available, it is utterly impossible for the medical physician to select the drugs he uses in the treatment of his patient wisely."

Statistics of the Yale-New Haven Hospital, which is associated with the Yale School of Medicine, showed five per cent of the hospital patients admissions were suffering from medication reactions. Extending these statistics to the 28 million hospital admissions in 1968, we find that nearly 1½ million people are hospitalized annually because of reactions to medications.

The Yale-New Haven statistics show that iatrogenic-caused diseases kill or contribute to the death of 100,000 Americans in hospitals each year. Adding complications and death from surgical error or faulty anesthesia, doctor and nurse error, doctor-caused deaths approximate 200,000 annually, close to cancer and heart disease as principal causes of death.

According to the *Medical World News*, June 18, 1965, Johns Hopkins University in Baltimore disclosed that approximately 14 per cent of its patients had drug reactions while hospitalized, some of which extended their stay and others that threatened their lives. Dr. Leighton Cluff, professor of medicine at Johns Hopkins University who conducted the study said, "Physicians ought to administer only those drugs that are critically necessary for the care of the patient. Improvement in therapeutics and control of dosage could reduce the problem."

DRUG ADDICTION

The most common form of drug addiction in America is tobacco smoking. In 1950 Drs. Evarts Grahem and Ernest Wynder of the St. Louis University School of Medicine studied 605 men with bronchogenic lung cancer (cancer originating in the bronchi of the lungs). They found that 96.5 per cent smoked at least one-half pack of cigarettes a day for 20 years. Only eight of the 605 cancer patients were nonsmokers. Such findings can be supported by a multitude of similar reports.

In 1970, an estimated 60,000 Americans died of lung cancer, a disease that is less frequent among nonsmokers.

A survey of over 40,000 doctors in England and Wales who quit smoking cigarettes revealed that the nonsmoker's death rate dropped by 38 per cent, while overall deaths from lung cancer in males actually had increased seven per cent.

American women today are smoking more than ever, and their average death rate from lung cancer is 400 per cent greater today than 40 years ago. The tragedy in women smoking lies in its effect upon the newborn child. Studies, which involved nine nations, concluded the following: Smoking women are more likely to have a stillborn baby or one that dies soon after birth. In Sheffield, England, a study of 2,000 pregnancies found the infant mortality rate almost twice as high. Children born to smoking mothers weighed a half pound less, were a half-inch shorter, were four months behind the average reading level for their age, were less adjusted to school environment, were clumsier, had an impaired spatial sense, and were among the lower 10 per cent in their class at copying drawings of simple designs. In short, the newborn were physically and mentally affected by the mother's smoking. The surgeon general's report also supported the statistics on lower birth weight and premature deliveries.

The adverse effect of smoking upon blood vessels is well established. Buerger's disease, a serious inflammatory condition of the arteries of the extremities, is one example. The disease is characterized by coldness, numbness, tingling, burning, weakness, and gangrene of the extremities. Buerger's disease is prevalent among smokers, and virtually nonexistent among nonsmokers.

The surgeon general report said that emphysema, characterized by a degeneration of the walls of the tiny air sacs in the lungs, is thirteen times more prevalent among smokers than among nonsmokers. This is very significant, since it is estimated that between one and ten million Americans are afflicted to some extent by the disease. The report, also said that smoking is the most important cause of chronic bronchitis in the United States, and that it increases the risk of dying from this condition.

The American Heart Association reports that the heart attack rate in heavy smokers was twice as high as in nonsmokers. In studies of various population groups, it found that death rates from heart attacks among male smokers ranged from 50 to 200 per cent higher than among nonsmokers.

Dr. Luther Terry, surgeon general of the U.S. Public Health Service, stated in 1965 in connection with deaths during a given year: "Studies of mortality rates of smokers and nonsmokers indicate 240,000 men will die prematurely from diseases associated with cigarette smoking . . . A reasonable estimate of excess deaths among women, added to the total of 240,000 for men, would bring the over-all total to 300,000. I consider this to be a reasonable estimate."

In 1967, the surgeon general, Dr. William Stewart, stated, too, that deaths due to smoking were in excess of 300,000 a year. If the surgeon general's report is correct, over 800 deaths a day in the United States can be attributed to cigarette smoking! Of these, 375 are due to diseases of the heart and circulation, 250 from bronchitis, emphysema, peptic ulcer and other diseases, and 175 from cancer.

Senator Frank Moss, speaking on the floor of the Senate in opposition to the federal subsidy of tobacco, said the United States was spending "millions and millions of dollars supporting the growth, export, advertising promotion and grading of this deadly plant." Senator Moss' staff estimated that the U.S. Agricultural Department annually spends $30 million in subsidies to encourage the export of tobacco, an additional $28 million in food and peace funds for foreign purchases, $6.5 million in administrative expenses connected with tobacco programs, $4.5 million for inspection and grading, $3.9 million in price supports, and $500,000 for advertising abroad.

Ironically, as we silently puff our lives away at the rate of 300,000 victims a year, more lives than we lost in all fronts of World War II, the federal government has been spending millions of dollars annually to subsidize this proven health hazard, while until 1974 it hasn't seen fit to spend one penny to subsidize the research and education of chiropractic, a profession which has contributed so much to the relief of human sickness and suffering. What a tragic testimonial to our ignorance and to our sense of values!

The subject of drug addiction brings up another widely discussed problem—drug abuse. In our drug-oriented society the pill is the "in" thing. It is socially acceptable and in some circles it is almost a status symbol. The "heavy sell" of drugs and self-medication has done much to promote and maintain this attitude. Although most doctors will agree that self-medication is not advisable, organized medicine does not exert the violent opposition to it that it does to so many other matters. After all, the AMA receives about one-half of its revenue from the pharmaceutical industry's advertisements in medical journals. Is it going to kick a gift horse in the mouth? As a result, persons with emotional problems, or adolescents going through the difficult phase of growing up, are being indoctrinated heavily on instant relief and pleasure. They soon rationalize that there are some drugs that will satisfy their emotional needs, after all, they can do everything else.

Thus we have come to grips with one of the most vicious and tragic evils of our time, drug abuse and addiction. President Nixon has referred to it as "Public enemy number one." The painful facts plague us as we read the newspapers, listen to the radio or watch television. We see the crippling and destroying of human lives with drugs, and live in the fear and hope that it will not some day strike one of our children or loved ones.

The concern over this situation was demonstrated by the March, 1971, issue of the *PTA Magazine*, the official national publication of the National Congress of Parents and Teachers. The front cover of this magazine emphasized a lead article entitled "Combating the Drug Peril" by William G. Hollister, M.D., director of the community psychiatry section in the school of medicine, University of North Carolina, and chairman of the National PTA Committee on Mental Health.

Dr. Hollister discussed some of the reasons why youths turn to drugs. He said: "Sensing the escape trend, the advertising industry uses it for commercial payoff. The message is that it is silly or stupid to endure adversities and rigorous living when we could escape to serenity through pill-popping and purchase of ease-giving, pleasure-giving products. Subtly we are taught that it is more modern and sophisticated to seek ease and pleasure than to endure reality, disappointment, and responsibility."

The *Chicago Today* on April 19, 1971, carried a review of the book, *You, Your Child and Drugs*. The book goes into a comprehensive study of the drug problem by the staff of the Child Study Association of America. This book quoted one 15-year-old boy as saying, "In my house you can't sneeze without getting a pill. My mother is always taking something for headaches and my father is always taking something to keep awake to get his work done at night. They're not drunks but they sure drink a lot. So now I'm a criminal for smoking pot?"

Another 13-year-old boy observed: "We're not supposed to take drugs but television is full of commercials showing people running for a pill because something is bugging them. All the magazines write it up (the drug problem) as if to warn you, but they go on about some rock star dying of an overdose of drugs and make it sound like something real groovy. It's not teenagers who are crazy. It's people."

The number of deaths in Cook County, Illinois, due to drug overdoses increased by 7,850 per cent in eight years, according to statistics kept by Cook County Coroner Andrew J. Toman. The drug overdose deaths rose from six in 1967 to an astounding 471 in 1975. And the trend is worsening. Dr. Toman said, "This is a crisis that is not confined to the inner city; it is also prevalent in our so called better neighborhoods. Drug abuse knows no economic, racial, social or ethnic limitations." Of the 471 drug deaths in 1975, 378 occurred in Chicago and 93 in the suburban area. He said 268 of the victims were white, 197 were black, two were oriental and four were American Indians.

As early as the 1950s the federal government could have enacted legislation to curb the illicit traffic of amphetamines and barbiturates, but failed because of opposition by medical and pharmaceutical associations. In fact, the AMA officially opposed the 1965 Drug Abuse Control Amendments.

A nationwide study of physicians was conducted by the Medical Disciplinary Committee of the AMA. Some of its conclusions were: "There is little apparent concern over such matters as narcotics addiction or fraud and deceit in practice. . . . Too often a 'guilty' physician is (merely) encouraged to go to another state. . . . There is failure on the part of individual physicians to recognize their responsibility in reporting ethical and professional violations. . . . The philosophy of present administrators of discipline . . . is very conservative and reluctant."

President Nixon, addressing the AMA convention on June 22, 1971, said that the nation is in danger of losing a whole generation to drugs. He said that many physicians are contributing to the drug problem by "prescribing drugs too often and too easily."

British police charge that overprescribing is the main cause of drug addiction in England. An overprescription bill was introduced in the British Parliament which would create a tribunal consisting of selected men of science, including doctors of medicine. Under the proposed bill complaints against a physician on the prescribing of drugs would be evaluated by this tribunal, and if adjudged guilty the doctor could be barred from writing specific drug prescriptions. Furthermore, a physician violating this ban would face a penalty of up to 14 years in prison. This is not to suggest that such extraordinary measures be instituted in this country; that is for the legislators to decide. It is intended rather to alert us to overprescribing as a major cause of drug abuse.

CONCLUSION

A physician's first obligation to his patient is to instruct the patient in the cause and prevention of disease. Too often the modern physician fails in this important duty and, instead, prescribes the appropriate medication for the symptom. The old proverb "An ounce of prevention is worth a pound of cure" applies very well here.

Proper dietary counseling is an important factor in health. Yet, 74 medical schools were surveyed and the finding was that no course on nutrition is offered in this vital area. Chiropractic colleges, on the other hand, offer an average of 54 hours on this important subject.

Hippocrates strongly advocated proper nutrition, the healing power of nature and minimum use of drugs. It is ironic then that the medical profession should adopt Hippocrates as its father of medicine, ask young men to repeat the Hippocratic oath on graduation, and yet fail to include a special course on nutrition in its medical schools.

It is easily recognized that we eat too much (often the wrong kind of food), smoke too much, and rely too heavily on escape and relief through indiscriminate use of drugs, rather than observe some of the natural laws of health.

Today, medicine generally concedes that it has been guilty of excessive use of surgery such as tonsillectomies, appendectomies and hysterectomies. It has admitted, supported by its own clinical observations, to excessive use of medications with iatrogenic reactions, and to excessive and indiscriminate use of antibiotics resulting in the development of more drug resistant bacterial organisms.

Ecology and pollution of our natural resources has been a topic of great concern and conversation in recent years. Yet, there is another form of ecology with which we must concern ourselves. It is the pollution of our body cells and fluids with the indiscriminate use of drugs. The way drug abuse, and drug addiction are taking place in this country, history should not only fully exonerate chiropractic's teachings, but prove it ecologically sound and deserving the highest respect among the healing arts. It also illustrates the need for a more rational utilization of both chiropractic and medicine.

CHAPTER XV

Chiropractic Recognition by American Medical Physicians

TO LIST all the American medical doctors who have supported the manipulative procedures, and even mentioned chiropractic by name, would be redundant. However the brief comments of a few of the nationally and internationally recognized authors, certified specialists and professors in the medical profession are as follows:

Dr. Charles Bechtol, chief of the orthopedic department at the University of California Los Angeles Medical Center, said, "I teach manipulations I learned from a professor who in turn learned them from what are called 'bonesetters' in England. Chiropractic has a place in the healing arts. The only quarrel we medical men have is that many chiropractors think theirs is the only art. Oddly enough, I found several medical practitioners who thought theirs, too, was the only art of healing!"

Louis Lasagna, M.D., nationally prominent professor of pharmacology at Johns Hopkins Medical School said, "Thousands of people utilize and are completely satisfied with the results of chiropractic, and that they (chiropractors) have as much, and perhaps more to offer." He added, "It is quite possible that organized medicine has overplayed its hand in denouncing them as cults."

B. Gomroe, M.D., faculty member at the University of Pennsylvania Medical School and a prominent author and lecturer, wrote in his book *Arthritis and Allied Conditions*: "They respond well to manipulative procedures. It is this type of patient who may be miraculously cured by certain mechanical maneuvers of chiropractors."

J. M. Nielsen, M.D., professor of neurology at the school of medicine, University of Southern California, and author of a widely read medical textbook entitled *Clinical Neurology*, discussed subluxations of lumbosacral and sacroiliac joints as a common cause of low back pain and attending sciatic neuralgia.

La Forest Potter, M.D., a New York orthopedic specialist, said that after practicing medicine for 15 years and using spinal adjustments for nearly 10, he was still astonished daily at the power of spinal adjustments as a cure for disease.

Philip Lewin, M.D., professor of bone and joint surgery of Northwestern University Medical School, spoke of backaches and minor errors and variations causing major discomforts and disabilities. In his book entitled *The Back and Its Disc Syndrome*, he said, "Postural backache is due to static errors resulting in muscular and ligamentous strain due to improper alignment. The spine is the seat of abnormalities that modify the normal mechanics, and predispose to stress, strain, weakness and disease."

Medical doctors, Braaf and Rosner, directors of the orthopedic and neurology departments at Stuyvesant Hospital in New York, studied 100 children with chronic headaches. They found that they all had headaches of the adult type without apparent cause. Scientists stretched their necks and produced lasting cures in 97 of them. The results of their investigation were reported in a story in the *Chicago Tribune* on May 7, 1970.

F. M. Pottenger, M.D., America's foremost authority on diseases of the internal organs and world renowned author of the textbook, *Symptoms of Visceral Diseases*, stated that diseases can be due to altered nerve activity.

Walter B. Cannon, M.D., professor of cardiology at Harvard University, is one of America's best known and respected cardiologists. He wrote in the *American Heart Journal* that nerves affect the state of the artery and bring about adaptions of vascular tone and change the flow of blood to the heart muscles. This is a significant fact in our battle against heart disease.

Ralph Soto Hall, M.D., one of America's most prominent orthopedists, stated that vertebral subluxations are the cause of many back problems and advocated manipulations for their correction.

Paul Ruegseggar, M.D., assistant professor of medicine at Cornell University Medical School, described treating "trigger points" around the neck in the treatment of headaches.

Louis Casamajor, M.D., professor of neurology at Columbia University, stated, "I have seen pain and illnesses of the human body which have been caused by subluxation or misalignment of the vertebrae. . . . There can be no doubt that the lumbar vertebrae, especially the fourth and fifth do slip back and forth at times, and when they slip out of alignment, they cause severe pain in the back and legs. This is relieved when they are put back in place."

Dr. Harold T. Hyman, associate professor of pharmacology at the College of Physicians and Surgeons of Columbia University, wrote in the *American Journal of Medical Science* in August, 1938, saying, "There is no doubt that the consciousness of the orthopedic surgeon was aroused originally by the success of the bonesetters, the early manipulators, and more recently the chiropractors . . . This latter group has undoubtedly performed its miraculous cures in individuals who have been misdiagnosed and mistreated by the practitioner or internist."

Jessie Wright, M.D., wrote a paper on the *Mechanics in Relation to Derangements of the Facet Joints of the Spine*, which was presented before the American Congress of Physical Therapy. He referred to vertebral subluxations resulting in pathologic change, altered body mechanics causing clinical symptoms and signs, and vertebral adjustments to restore articular surfaces to normal relationship.

Lee Hadley, M.D., a renowned author, lecturer, and senior roentgenologist at Syracuse Memorial Hospital, wrote of subluxation and resultant encroachment upon the vertebral foramina in the *American Journal of Roentgenology.*

Neville T. Ussher, M.D., conducted extensive work with the research department of the Santa Barbara Clinic. In the May, 1940, issue of *Annals of Internal Medicine,* following 15 years of clinical study, he reported a direct connection between visceral conditions and spinal distortions. He purposely did not tell any patients that he was adjusting their spine to correct any visceral condition because he wanted to completely eliminate any possibility of psychosomatic suggestion. Without using any drugs he manipulated the spine and corrected 400 visceral conditions, he said in the article.

Dr. John M. Mennell, chief of physical medicine at Brentwood Veterans Hospital in Los Angeles, associate professor of physical medicine and rehabilitation at the University of Pennsylvania and University of Southern California School of Medicine, and author of the book *Back Pain,* counsels doctors that under certain circumstances "I think you are justified in asking a well trained manipulator, whoever he may be, to treat your patient for that specific complaint, just as you would ask . . . a pharmacist to make up a prescription . . . Do not deprive your patients of relief from pain because of your prejudices."

Edward L. Compere, M.D., is one of Chicago's most renowned orthopedic surgeons. In response to the question, "Is it possible to manipulate spinal vertebrae by hand to relieve underlying pathology?" Dr. Compere said:

"Many orthopedists as well as osteopaths have demonstrated that it is possible to manipulate the spinal vertebrae by hand and relieve pressure on nerve roots. The exact nature of the lesion which responds to this type of manipulation has never been fully established. In all probability in the case of subluxations or slight slippage of the articular facet in a spine where the neural foramina may be narrowed by osteophyte formation or because of edema of the surrounding tissue, manipulation may readjust the articular process sufficiently to relieve pressure on the nerve. I have personally relieved patients who were in severe pain by a manipulation intended to loosen up tension on articular facets of the spine, or to restore a normal anatomic relationship between vertebral bodies, so that there is no longer an impingement on a nerve root. Exactly what is accomplished by these manipulations no one has fully explained. The fact that they do definitely relieve some of these patients, especially those who have had their back pain or sciatica for a short time, cannot be denied. Anyone who is familiar with the simple manipulative procedures which are usually carried out should try them before resorting to more definitive procedures."

Dr. Compere's comments were printed in the December 24, 1960 issue of the *JAMA*. Somehow, this type of information never seems to be found in *Today's Health*, the AMA magazine which is frequently found in the waiting room of the medical doctor.

A study of the effects of chiropractic care was conducted by members of the Kentucky College of Medicine. The 18 month study was supported in part by the Kentucky Medical Association and the U.S. Public Health Service. Appearing in the Journal of the Kentucky Medical Association under the authorship of Richard Park, B.S., Jessie W. Tapp, M.D., and D. L. Hochstrasser, Ph.D., it said: "Undoubtedly, many patients with functional complaints feel better after the personal and manipulative attention of a chiropractor. Furthermore, it appears that some patients suffering from chronic or obscure complaints turn to chiropractors after failing to secure the type of relief they expected from doctors of medicine. . . ."

Perhaps the most widely used and respected physician's

desk reference book in America is the *Merck Manual.* The first edition of this reference book was issued in 1899 and has been periodically updated and revised. Among authors of this reference book are more than 100 outstanding clinicians from America and Europe. The book is reviewed by an editorial board and by special consultants.

In regard to sciatica, the 1950 *Merck Manual* frankly admitted, "Some physicians have reported good results with manipulative procedures with or without anesthesia." Regarding headaches, the 1966 *Merck Manual* said, "Headaches may result from stimulation or traction of or pressure on, any pain sensitive structures of the head . . . and upper cervical nerves."

MEDICAL ECONOMICS

The July 19, 1971 issue of *Medical Economics* printed an 11 page article on chiropractic, complete with pictures and illustrations. It was based on observations by the author while visiting a chiropractor's office. The article provided chiropractic case histories, professional men and businessmen, whom the author met and interviewed in this chiropractic office. The histories showed how patients rejected medical recommendations for hospitalization, surgery, bed rest, traction, back braces, and other procedures and turned, though sometimes reluctantly, to chiropractic and received relief from a number of conditions including sciatica, tension, back injuries, headaches and asthma.

This article is very significant since *Medical Economics* is a publication written exclusively for the medical physician, and *Medical Economics* specified that the article could not be reproduced, quoted or paraphrased in whole or in part in any manner whatsoever without the written permission of the copyright owner. Of course, permission to use the article by the chiropractic profession was denied, and the public was withheld these privileged facts. But why deprive the public of the truth?

Medical Economics did not print this article as an endorsement of chiropractic. Indeed, the article was preceded by a foreword which repeated a condemnation of chiropractic made five years earlier by *Medical Economics.*

Why, then, did *Medical Economics* publish the article? It did so in an attempt to give medical doctors some hints on how chiropractic works after a medical doctor has failed. It was, in effect, a warning to medical doctors that they ought to do more than they are doing for their patients.

The *Medical Economics* article backfired when Senator Quentin N. Burdick from North Dakota entered it into the *Congressional Record* on June 16, 1972. This made the article public record! Nevertheless, the chiropractic profession was restrained from using the record.

The *Congressional Record* of November 18, 1971, carries a statement of Congressman Henry Helstoski from New Jersey made before the House of Representatives. It is entitled, "Medical Research Proves Chiropractic." In the statement he quoted medical research supporting the value of chiropractic, and urged medicine to accept the proof of its own research. He also provided several testimonials of individuals who had been helped through chiropractic care, and said: "There is no argument with a cured case, regardless of the method used. In view of statistics from both medical and chiropractic research, isn't it logical that medical doctors and chiropractors should work more closely together for better health for everyone? . . . When the patient leaves the chiropractor's office, with all or part of his pain removed, he knows that chiropractic works . . . and so do millions of Americans who seek chiropractic care every year."

CHAPTER XVI

Chiropractic Recognition in Other Countries

A FEW prominent medical physicians, along with their country origin, are given with their comments:

GERMANY

Nearly 1,500 German medical physicians participated in a mammoth project to examine the scientific validity and basis for chiropractic. They concluded that "CHIROPRACTIC IS SCIENTIFICALLY WELL FOUNDED, IS ONE OF THE MOST EFFECTIVE NEUROTHERAPEUTIC MEASURES KNOWN, AND BELONGS IN THE VERY CENTER OF MEDICINE."

The results of the study were published in the German medical journal *Hippokrates* in February, 1956, August, 1957, September, 1957, and April, 1958.

On December 12, 1953, the Medical Research and Cooperative Society for Chiropractic was formed by 80 prominent independent physicians in Hamburg, Germany. By 1958, the membership increased to 347 members. After years of research, scientific analysis and laboratory experiments, they released four reports, which were later translated to English.

The four reports were as follows: *Chiropractic as a Rational Medical Therapy*, by G. Gutmann, M.D.; a report by Professor K. R. von Roques concluding, "Chiropractic as a neurotherapeutic measure belongs in the very center of medicine"; another report, *Functional Changes of the Diencephalon (mid-brain) Through Manipulative Vertebral Therapy*, by A. H. Sollmann, professor of surgery, Munich, Germany, and finally, *Fundamentals of Chiropractic from a Standpoint of a Medical Doctor*, by Freimut Biedermann, M.D.

Dr. Biedermann showed great wisdom and truth in his report when he wrote: "We medical doctors who have studied and used chiropractic techniques and have proven its indisputable value cannot understand the negative attitude of medicine towards chiropractic. . . . Coming from the ranks of traditional medicine myself, and being familiar with its principles and therapeutic methods, I have learned well to evaluate its necessity and merit for the sick. However, having learned rather extensively for several years the chiropractic teachings and after practicing chiropractic more and more, I do know also, that the healing art chiropractic has its indisputable merits, and that it is worthy of, and deserves to be used in, the care of the sick. It does not enter my mind to play the role of an umpire between chiropractic and traditional medicine. I intend only to make a breach in the wall of ignorance and prejudice, which still widely separates both healing arts. This wall has to be broken down by both parties. For the sake of the sick we must understand each other and join hands. If my exposition only stimulates both sides for better mutual understanding, then I will have obtained my goal."

Dr. Gutmann's report, *Chiropractic as Rational Medical Therapy*, provided a statistical chart showing his results with low back pain under spinal manipulative care. He used exceptionally stubborn cases which were unresponsive to baths, massage, novocaine injections, disc operations, and other procedures. He found that after two or three chiropractic adjustments, 77 per cent of the patients were either relieved or much improved. And that in none of the cases were back braces or supports used.

Dr. Gutmann wrote: "On the basis of our experience over the years, we believe that we may declare that many costly and time consuming tests, many treatments adding up in time to high costs, periods spent in clinic or sanitarium, and certainly lawsuits of years' duration would become superfluous, if the manipulative vertebral therapy called chiropractic were exactly applied."

It should be emphasized here that a chiropractic adjustment is not a massage. Rather, it is a carefully planned, properly executed, specific movement of vertebrae designed to restore mobility of the joints, and allow the vertebrae to assume proper functional relationship with each other. Dr. Gutmann's study and observations clearly indicated that the cases in which "massage was ineffective" were dramatically responsive to a specifically executed chiropractic adjustment. Critics of chiropractic frequently have confused this point by comparing a chiropractic adjustment to a massage. In so doing they exhibit gross ignorance on the subject.

Dr. Gutmann reported in *Hippokrates*, August 31, 1957, "We have been permitted in certain cases unsuccessfully treated for years, even for decades, to demonstrate the usefulness of chiropractic." In *Neuralmedizin* in May, 1953, he reported his success with 2,000 patients with cervical (neck) problems, saying, "I could not find in all the medical literature a single contribution of equal importance with respect to the problems herein discussed."

Dr. Sollmann's report stated, "The extraordinary experiences which have been obtained with so many a vertebral manipulative therapy and the changes in the health of people which have been obtained through this therapy have prompted us to search deeper into the cause of these phenomena."

Drs. Sollmann and Worner reporting in *Hippokrates*, on

August 31, 1956, said, "In these researches on 150 patients, noteworthy results were shown which we believe it is our duty to report. . . . Summing up, we would draw from this sample of the most thoroughly studied patients the following conclusion: According to the most stringent medical—and, in our case surgical—indications, the answer to the question as to whether there is or not a vertebral therapeutic influence on serologically proved events, is yes."

K. R. von Roques, M.D., wrote an article that appeared in *Neuralmedizin*, June, 1954, in which he said, "We must recognize—insofar as we have been concerned therewith—that many ailments or diseases are enormously accelerated in their improvement by spinal therapy; indeed many a cure thereby becomes possible for the first time."

L. Zukschwerdt, M.D., professor of surgery at the University of Hamburg, wrote in *Neuralmedizin* in May, 1953: "Chiropractic offers medicine substantial material with which to busy itself in the years to come . . . I would beg you not to neglect the application of so worthwhile a method for the practicing physician." In his introduction to a medical book he wrote, "The acute intervertebral disc, a particular form of the chiropractic subluxation, gave me the first understanding for the possibility of the chiropractic adjustment."

Drs. Kemlin et al., in *Hippokrates*, on September 15, 1957, said, In the light of Gutzeit's researches it does not appear so wrong . . . that loss of appetite, headache, dizziness, insomnia, and heart sensations may be treated through the spine."

Dr. A. A. Hochfeld, in *Zeitschrift für Arztliche Fortbildung*, a journal of medical education, said, "Chiropractic is thoroughly suited to be accorded an authorized place in our therapy chest . . . Experienced and critical observers of chiropractic . . . see in it a substantial enrichment of our present methods of treatment and treasure it because sometimes, under a practicing chiropractor, it gives astonishing success quickly and painlessly." The article appeared on November 1, 1956.

Albert Cramer, M.D., studied the results of chiropractic on 6,000 patients over a four year period. In a textbook on the subject he concluded that chiropractic is a "necessity of our civilization." Writing in the medical journal, *Hippokrates*, on November 2, 1955, he said, "The great possibilities of chiropractic lie in the exactly purposeful removal of the spinal dynamics."

Dr. Gutzeit, a highly respected German clinician, wrote a paper, *The Spine as Causative Factor of Disease*, in which he published the findings of his clinical research. Some of the conditions he attributed to change in the spine were cerebrovascular disturbances of vasomotor character, vertebral subluxations with loss of appetite, headaches, dizziness, insomnia, heart sensations and gastrointestinal changes. He said that the viscera also suffered functional disturbances, histological damage, and changes in its structural make-up.

Karl Sell, M.D., chief of staff of the Orthopedic Hospital at Allagan, addressed 5,000 medical physicians at the German Therapy Week Convention in 1953 at Karlsruhe. He spoke enthusiastically of the merits of chiropractic and was met the following day by a long line of medical doctors waiting to receive personal chiropractic adjustments from him. The story of this convention, and of the medical doctors lining up for adjustments, was published in *Der Spiegel*, the German equivalent of *Time Magazine*.

Hans Kusche, M.D., wrote in *Hippokrates*, September 15, 1957: "Internists, roentgenologists, neurologists, orthopedists, and gynecologists are all concerned with the diagnosis and therapy of spinal trouble. The results of their efforts have not been very encouraging; otherwise it would be hard to understand how chiropractic has taken such an upswing. The success of manual therapy cannot be discussed away . . . Medicines are of subordinate importance, because by their very nature they can work only symptomatically."

RUSSIA

Dr. A. D. Speransky, director of the department of pathophysiology of the All Union Institute of Experimental Medicine in Leningrad, conducted extensive documented research on the nervous system's role in health. He published books on his 10 year research with live animals. He was able to produce visceral dysfunction and disease in laboratory animals by altering their nerve function. His conclusion was that normal nerve integrity is essential for maintaining body health and that faulty nerve function can cause many pathological changes. He wrote: "Many pathological processes, the cause of which have been regarded as absolutely foreign to nervous influence, have been found to be in reality entirely dependent on the latter for their origin. To whatever chapter of pathology pathological processes belong, however complicated their composition and however variable their course, the nervous component remains from beginning to end the factor that determines their general state."

ENGLAND

The First Congress of International Federation of Manual Medicine met in London in 1968. It brought together hundreds of medical physicians from all parts of the world, enthusiastic in the manipulative procedures in healing. Its expressed purpose was then and is still to study, teach, research and advance the manipulative procedures under the banner of medicine. Also, the British Medical Association recognizes spinal manipulation as part of its medicine.

Edgar Cyriax, M.D., one of England's outstanding neurologists, said: "In the course of time I have seen 1,000 cases of minor displacements of the vertebrae, and I have become convinced that in certain proportion of the cases the malposition present was wholly or partially responsible for numerous symptoms, whether visceral or nonvisceral."

R. S. Henderson, M.D., wrote in the *British Medical Journal* in September 13, 1952, about his clinical research with 500 patients at the department of orthopedics, St. Bartholomew Hospital, in England. He treated 129 cases solely with extension exercises and achieved good results in 90 per cent of the cases.

James Mennell, M.D., England's world renowned orthopedist and author of the book, *The Science and Art of Joint Manipulation*, wrote: "It is indisputable that the testimony is overwhelming that countless patients have derived relief from aches and pains of a great variety as a result of manipulation of the joints of the back. This is only what we should expect once we realize that the joints in question are just as much joints in every detail as are those of the extremities. The only difference is that, from the very nature of their shape and movement and the stresses that are laid upon them, they are more liable to 'lock' with the creation of a 'lesion.' Local pain would thus be caused, and relief would reasonably be expected to follow manipulative treatment if properly applied in suitable cases. . . . It is thus that many patients claim, and quite rightly, the cure of widespread symptoms as the result of spinal manipulation."

James Henry Cyriax, M.D., an outstanding British orthopedic surgeon, is considered one of the world's prominent authorities on the backache. Lecturing before the California Medical Association's 100th annual scientific session on conservative therapy for backache he said, "It's a crying shame that more physicians are not interested in manipulation of the spine to solve backache problems, because that technique, properly done, could save an awful lot of surgery bills." Later, at a press conference, he said, "My experience, based on more than 40,000 backache cases, has shown that one per cent or fewer need surgery and 52 per cent can be cured by one session of manipulation."

Philip Wiles, M.D., also a British orthopedic surgeon, discussed in detail the many merits of spinal manipulation techniques for the treatment of back pain, in his widely read textbook, *Essentials of Orthopedics.* As do chiropractors, Dr. Wiles referred to "spinal subluxations" as source of back pain.

John F. Bourdillon, M.D., British orthopedic surgeon and author of the textbook *Spinal Manipulation*, wrote: "The very success of the osteopaths and the chiropractors should be a stimulus to the orthodox medical profession to undertake an unbiased assessment of their ideas, methods and claims by those competent to do so . . . So far most such investigations have been conducted in a thoroughly unscientific manner and started with a strong bias against the subject under investigation."

Correcting deafness, tinnitus (ear ringing) and dizziness through spinal manipulation, Dr. Bourdillon made reference to Dr. Palmer's similar success with deafness. He wrote: "The claim, however, may not be quite as fantastic as it sounds . . . When the thoracic spine was examined, the lesion at T 4-5 joint was found and manipulative treatment to this joint resulted in dramatic and lasting relief of all symptoms referred to, including the deafness."

CANADA

Chiropractic has been growing rapidly in Canada. In the 1930s, it was licensed in Alberta, Ontario and British Columbia. Today it is also licensed and recognized in Manitoba, Saskatchewan, New Brunswick, and Prince Edward Island, and it is included in the national health program.

A royal commission in Quebec conducted a study which said that chiropractic is a valuable method of treatment and should be available to the people of Quebec. The commission said that chiropractors are not dangerous, as charged by medical doctors, and are qualified to diagnose and treat patients. They commended the Canadian Memorial Chiropractic College for its high educational standards. The commission recommended that chiropractic legislation be enacted to regulate its practice. And it warned medical doctors not to obstruct this legislation as such action would not be in the interest of the public.

In July, 1970, the Canadian Medical Association amended its code of ethics to allow an ethical physician to "cooperate with those individuals who, in the opinion of the physicians, may assist in the care of the patient." The new code permits the Canadian medical physicians to refer their patients to a chiropractor. Many chiropractors have reported a significant improvement in interprofessional cooperation since that time.

W. B. Parsons, M.D., wrote about chiropractic in the Canadian Medical Journal: "The reason we took up manipulation was an interest in backache, with the early discovery that many patients who failed to respond to routine medical treatment went to a manipulator and received immediate relief." He concluded the article with the classic advice, " 'If you can't whip 'em, join 'em,' at least to the extent of borrowing their technique."

R. A. Leeman, M.D., wrote an article in the journal of the Canadian Medical Association on April 1, 1958, entitled *Pain Syndromes Originating in the Vertebral Column and their Amenability to Manipulative Treatment.* In reviewing the article, the journal said: "The addition of chiropractic maneuvers to general management permits treatment of the cause rather than effect." The journal also noted that involvement of the sympathetic nerve fibers may produce circulatory and dystrophic disturbances.

A few years ago, during a meeting of the Ontario Medical Association, its president, W. J. S. Melvin, M.D., announced: "With the growing interest in manipulation for back pain, the doctor of chiropractic seems to be in a favorable position, since there is no doubt he is better at manipulation than most doctors . . . Chiropractors do not make people worse, they make an awful lot of people an awful lot better."

DENMARK

Paul Bechgaard, M.D., professor of internal medicine at the University of Aarhus, wrote that a patient with a chronic hearing defect, unsuccessfully treated by an ear specialist for seven years, was aided by receiving spinal manipulation for lumbago. This prompted him to manipulate other patients with hearing defects, and he obtained good results in six cases. His conclusions were based on auditory (hearing) tests before and after manipulation. He also found that impaired blood supply to the ear (organ of Corti) was the cause of the hearing defect brought on by irritated sympathetic nerves from the upper thoracic spine. His article was published in *Nordisk Medicine* on June 6, 1963.

Dr. Bøze, the senior physician at Rigshospital, Copenhagen, and lecturer in physical medicine at the university medical school, wrote in the publication of the Danish Medical Association in 1956: "Manipulative treatment, which previously in this country was given exclusively by chiropractors, has in later years been taken up by some physicians, among others, the writer, who has found that this therapy is of significant value. . . . It must be emphasized that it requires great clinical experience and great technical skill to perform these manipulations. . . . As for my opinion, such a difficult form of therapy ought to be given by physicians who have specialized in this field and mastered the technique to perfection. . . . Manipulative treatment cannot be considered equivalent to massage and therapeutic exercise which may justifiably be carried out by assistants. . . . If the physiotherapists want to use manipulative treatment, they ought to get an education just as thorough as that of chiropractors."

SWITZERLAND

H. De Brunner, M.D., professor of orthopedics, school of medicine, University of Basel, testified before a government commission, saying: "The attitude of clinical medicine toward chiropractic has radically changed within the last few years. In the mid-1930s, it was denounced in our country. Today, however, many medical doctors are in favor of chiropractic and consider it to be an excellent therapeutic measure for certain diseases having their origin in changes within the spinal column."

J. Terrier, M.D., specialist in rheumatology in Baden, Switzerland, wrote in Bulletin des Medecins Suisses No. 9, 1959: "It could be truly incomprehensible and unjustifiable to continue to exclude chiropractors. . . . from commissions concerned with public health."

FRANCE, AUSTRIA, AUSTRALIA

Charles M. Rocher, M.D., wrote in the *Bordeaux Chirurgical* in October, 1952: "The 600 cases we observed over four years have taught us superabundantly that vertebrotherapy constitutes important currency in the changing gamut of means to combat diverse pains in the vertebral sphere, and it often constitutes the only means of curing, and that in a manner which is at times spectacular . . . The manipulations extolled by the chiropractor are multiple and varied, but do not concern back pain only."

Adolph Lorenz, M.D., son of the world famous Viennese surgeon, described spinal manipulation as "a blessed substitute for the usual reparatory methods."

Gordon Rich, M.D., writing in the *Australian Medical Journal*, said: "It has always been recognized by some medical practitioners that a minor degree of dislocation known as subluxation, as distinct from luxation or complete dislocation, can and does occur. Subluxation of the sacroiliac joint is a well established entity, but in this paper I wish to draw attention to subluxations occurring in the cervical spine particularly."

R. J. Berry, M.D., dean of the faculty of medicine, University of Melbourne, and author of the book, *Brain and*

Mind, wrote, "There can be no disease which does not disturb the nerve cells concerned; hence it is important for these conducting nerve paths to be studied from the modern standpoint of the ingoing (receptor) nerve impulses and outgoing or (effector) ones. If the cause of the disturbance of these conducting nerves can be ascertained or removed, the patient will be cured. If not, treatment merely diverts from the truth."

Dr. Maitland, medical physician and instructor in physiotherapy at the University of Adelaide, applauded the manipulative approach to healing in his book, *Vertebral Manipulation.*

JAPAN

Manipulative therapy has been practiced for centuries in Japan. Although chiropractic in Japan is not as sophisticated as in America, a growing enthusiasm for this method has become evident.

In July, 1971, a study group consisting of about sixty Japanese health officials, medical orthopedists, osteopaths and chiropractors toured various chiropractic facilities in the United States, and attended chiropractic seminars and workshops.

The purpose of the study group, as explained by one of the doctors, "is to take a first hand view of the advance of chiropractic in the United States which we hope will aid us in our plans to develop chiropractic in Japan."

OTHER COUNTRIES

Chiropractic or spinal manipulative procedures are recognized and practiced in more countries than those already mentioned. Among them are Scandinavia, Poland, Italy, Africa, South America, New Zealand, Belgium, Ireland, and India. In fact, some form of manipulative therapy is practiced in nearly every country in the world.

CHAPTER XVII

Chiropractic Research

THE late Bernard Baruch, famous philanthropist and statesman, in 1943, made a grant of $1,100,000 to study the physical methods of treatment. In 1944, the results of that study concluded, "There is a definite need for careful study of the various manipulative procedures which are employed therapeutically to alter the structure mechanics of the human body."

In spite of the conclusion of the Baruch report and the national and international recognition and research documenting the validity of chiropratic, the federal government had never financially supported any chiropractic research or educational program until 1974, even though the government had been spending $400 million a year for medical research through the National Institute of Health under the U.S. Public Health Service.

The International Chiropractors Association initiated a chiropractic research study entitled, "Bioengineering Analysis of Spinal Systems," at the University of Colorado. Its principal investigators are Ronald J. MacGregor, Ph.D., and Chung-Ha Suh, Ph.D. The research focuses upon computer-aided x-ray analysis, computer graphics for studying biometrics of the spine, and development of general computational models for studying electrical activity in large groups of interconnected neurons. The project was instrumental in obtaining for chiropractic a $2 million governmental appropriation, and indicated the beginning of an era of governmental subsidation of chiropractic research. By 1976 the ICA had contributed nearly a quarter of a million dollars to the project. Also the Foundation for Chiropractic Education and Research spent about one-third of a million dollars on research projects in chiropractic colleges and other colleges and universities, and increased its research commitments for the coming years.

INSTITUTE FOR THE STUDY OF THE MECHANICS, STATICS AND DYNAMICS OF THE HUMAN BODY

The director of the Institute for the Study of the Mechanics, Statics and Dynamics of the Human Body for the European Chiropractic Union is Dr. F. W. Illi of Switzerland. His research included a study of the body mechanics in all positions, including walking, standing, flexion and extension. Much information already has been compiled and catalogued. He originated new techniques in the use of x-ray motion pictures (cineroentgenology) of the human spine and pelvis in action. He was able to prove, through the use of these motion pictures, that the sacroiliac joint is a movable joint and that it influences compensatory changes throughout the spinal column. He disproved previous theories held by the medical profession that the sacroiliac joint was immovable.

An American chiropractor, Dr. Earl Rich, also conducted spinal x-ray motion pictures. He proved that all component parts of joint action are integrated and dependent, one upon the other.

NERVE COMPRESSION AND DISEASE

The neurological effect of compression subluxations can be demonstrated by numerous medical, chiropractic, and osteopathic authorities. A few contemporary ones include medical researchers Weiss and Hiscoe, chiropractic researcher Haldeman, and osteopathic researcher Cole. The effects of nerve compression were carried out on test animals. Nerves were cut free, stimuli were applied, and oscilloscopic observations were made of the effects of mechanical pressure on the nerves. Microscopic studies of the nerves, before and after nerve compression, were recorded. Microscopically, bulging and swelling of the nerve axon proximal to the side of compression was noted. Also, the flow of axoplasm (neural fluid) was obstructed with a "damming up" of its vital constituents. Consequently, nerve impulses were unable to pass the compressed area, proving that nerve conduction can be blocked mechanically. Microscopic studies also showed that the removal of the mechanical compression on the nerves resulted in restoration of nerve function. Where mechanical compression was sustained for a longer period, however, fibrous adhesions occurred at the site of compression causing irreversible damage.

Dr. Cole, studying the visceral effects of nerve compression, created artificial vertebral fixations or "subluxations" on test animals. He did this by injecting chemicals, using electrical stimuli, and tying vertebrae together. By fixating or subluxating the vertebrae neurologically associated with the liver, heart or kidney, he was able to create pathological changes in these viscera which were documented microscopically. Indeed, chiropractic's premise of vertebral subluxation, nerve conduction block, and visceral pathology was clearly demonstrated.

DEPARTMENT OF RESEARCH AND STATISTICS

The department of research and statistics was established in Glendale, California, in 1959, with Henry Higley, M.S., D.C., of Alhambra, California, as its director. The facilities and staff are composed of faculty members from cooperating chiropractic colleges. By using the facilities of these colleges, they are able to stay within a limited budget. The purpose of the department is to act as a clearing house for research information, assist and encourage colleges in various projects, conduct investigations into the mechanics of the human body and related structures, and to serve as consultants in research methodology. In 1960 the department completed a study, "The Intervertebral Disc Syndrome," which went into a study of the disc, and its progress through treatment. The monograph was well-received by scientific groups and copies were requested and sent to government agencies. It also was reviewed in the *Biometrics* journal which deals with the mathematical and statistical aspects of biology, and in *Index Medicus*, which is the official publication of the National Library of Medicine.

OTHER RESEARCH PROJECTS

Some of the research studies presently conducted or completed at chiropractic colleges are as follows:

Controlled clinical studies of the effects of exercise upon patients with and without chiropractic adjustments.

Dissection studies to determine intervertebral discopathy due to gravitational stress.

Radiographic analysis of tortipelvis, intervertebral disc modifications and vertebral orthodiarthria.

Evaluation of vertebral facet facings.

Static and kinetic juxta-positional vertebral mensuration and cineradiography.

The effects of chiropractic therapy in the treatment of multihandicapped children.

Postural study of junior and senior high school students.

Correlation of clinical syndromes with anatomy and physiology of the nervous system.

CONCLUSION

The chiropractic profession supports expanded research within its profession. In the survey of 6,000 chiropractors, conducted by Batten and Associates in 1962, 92.5 per cent supported the need for greater chiropractic research. Six and one-half per cent offered no opinion while only one per cent rejected the need.

The federal government and foundations contribute millions for medical research, while the chiropractic profession must completely subsidize its own research. This places an unreasonable economic burden upon the chiropractic profession. Although organized medicine exerts every effort to discourage governmental financial aid for chiropractic research, it supports the false charge: "Not a single shred of scientific proof has been furnished . . . not a shred of scientific evidence exists to prove the Palmer theory." Indeed, volumes of scientific and clinical proof does exist. The last three chapters have demonstrated a few examples.

CHAPTER XVIII

Prominent People Support Chiropractic

MANY notable people throughout the world have received chiropractic care. They include presidents and vice-presidents of the United States, congressmen, governors, professional men and women, movie stars, and prominent businessmen.

Eleanor Roosevelt, wife of the 32nd President, once said: "There are certain things I do regularly, a once-a-month visit to the dentist, the chiropractor, and the family chiropodist (podiatrist)."

One of the remaining giants of the movie industry is John Wayne, an enthusiastic supporter of chiropractic. There is perhaps no more loved or respected movie idol in the country today.

Thomas A. Edison, one of America's greatest inventors, was a patient, and a firm supporter of chiropractic. He once said: "The doctor of the future will give no medicine, but will interest his patients in the care of the human frame, in diet, and in the cause and prevention of disease."

"Rocky" Marciano had been ailing with a back condition early in his boxing career. Medical orthopedic specialists advised him that he needed spinal surgery. Of course, his boxing career appeared finished. Turning to chiropractic care, his back ailment was not only corrected, but he went on to become the heavyweight boxing champion of the world. During speaking engagements, he frequently expressed his gratitude and enthusiasm toward chiropractic.

Another great athlete that had his career saved through chiropractic was baseball star Roberto Clemente. Back in 1957, he was benched for a neck ailment and ready to quit baseball. Turning to chiropractic, he had his condition corrected, and resumed an active and brilliant career.

Mr. Melvin Belli, one of America's most renowned defense lawyers, had chronic headaches for 32 years. After extensive medical care without relief, he turned to chiropractic, and rid himself of the headaches.

Mr. Belli had this to say about chiropractic: "The only practitioners I've found who seem to have any success in diminishing the agony of whiplash are chiropractors. I'm not completely sure what they do with their magic fingers, but somehow they have helped me and countless others I know who have suffered from this traumatic condition. All I know is that after medical specialists, including learned neurologists, from Boston to San Francisco, had cracks at me and fed me so many tranquilizers that I began to doze in court, chiropractors were the only ones who managed to alleviate my chronic headaches."

Today, enthusiastically and intensely dedicated to chiropractic, Mr. Belli says that chiropractic has given him a "reprieve" and a new life without pain.

Lawrence Welk's Champagne Lady, Norma Zimmer, and her family have received remarkable help from chiropractic through the years. Most recently, Mrs. Zimmer feared that numbness of her face, arm and leg might prove disabling and prevent her from continuing her work with the Lawrence Welk show. Turning again to chiropractic she was able to overcome her condition and remain with the show.

Patrick McGoohan, producer and star of two television

series, "Secret Agent" and "The Prisoner," made the following statement on chiropractic in the November, 1972 issue of *Chiropractic Economics*:

"I was personally saved from spinal surgery through the benefits of the profession. My eldest daughter was given at best a life in a wheelchair; she has now been restored to such health and vitality that she is herself studying to be a doctor of chiropractic."

McGoohan's dedication to chiropractic is reflected in his plan to direct a chiropractic documentary movie which he hopes will ". . . destroy for all time this ignorance and prejudice and to show the world the true concept of a profound natural healing force."

Football star Fred Cox of the Minnesota Vikings had suffered for 10 years with a chronic back ailment. After receiving chiropractic care, he was so impressed with the help he received that he enrolled in a chiropractic college and became a chiropractor.

Singer John Gary collapsed with acute back pain during a performance. He was taken to a hospital and after three weeks of extensive examinations, spinal traction and medical treatment, was advised by doctors that back surgery was necessary. Mr. Gary balked at the idea of surgery, leaving the hospital under medical protest. He went to a Los Angeles chiropractor who eliminated the pain and enabled him to continue a 1966 summer replacement television series which was vital to his professional career. In an interview six years later, Mr. Gary revealed that his back had never felt better, and that he had no recurrence of the prior condition.

John D. Rockefeller, Sr., received regular chiropractic care until his death at the age of 98. Following his death in 1937, the family sent his chiropractor a telegram which said, "The family joins me in sincere appreciation of your wonderful help and splendid service during the years you have treated the distinguished patient."

James Arness, the towering marshal in the "Gunsmoke" television series, had a whiplash injury and found relief through chiropractic after everything else had failed.

Jeanne Dixon, nationally famous psychic, also received personal help through chiropractic care. A grateful and enthusiastic supporter of chiropractic, she views it as a rising star in the horizon.

The Bob Cromie Column in the *Chicago Tribune* on March 18, 1971, carried the headline, "Chiropractor Saves Dance Star." It began: "Erik Bruhn, regarded by many as the world's greatest male dancer, is back in town with the American Ballet Theater. . . . And you can thank a Danish chiropractor for Bruhn's presence."

The article went on to explain that Mr. Bruhn had been ailing with an acutely painful neck. Numerous medical specialists were unable to correct the condition. After eight months of pain, which prevented him from dancing, he turned to chiropractic. The results were dramatic and immediate. He walked from the chiropractor's office without pain and was able to resume professional dancing.

The late Andrew J. Sordoni of Pennsylvania, a director of 14 corporations including a utility company, several telephone companies, six hotels and thousands of acres of farmland, provided his thousands of employees with chiropractic care. Sordoni, who was also a member of the Pennsylvania senate wrote: "Medical doctors, surgeons and chiropractors all have their specific attributes. Each must work hand-in-hand with each other . . . these sciences do not conflict, but rather, supplement each other. . . . insurance companies . . . state workmen's compensation acts are more and more recognizing the need for chiropractic services. These bodies form their decisions and base their policies on statistics, not on sentiment. Through chiropractic, they've realized tremendous savings. I personally have experienced its marvelous benefits and have seen the magnificent role it can play in industry. I have seen it save suffering, needless loss of time, money, and health.

Chiropractic in industry will continue to win an ever-widening recognition, for it makes the lives of all those it touches happier, more productive, and more meaningful."

One of the March of Dimes polio models was five year old Winifred Gardella of Stockton, California. Large reproductions of her picture were used during the 1952–53 March of Dimes Campaign. It showed her in a hospital crib and carried the following caption:

> WILL WALK AGAIN . . .
>
> Little Winifred, lying on her stomach reading a comic book, doesn't appear to have a care in the world. A victim of polio, her chances of complete recovery have been enhanced by March of Dimes. Hundreds like Winifred are dependent for future care on the March of Dimes campaign.

The irony of all this is that Winifred was declared a "hopeless paraplegic" after 2½ years direct care of the National Foundation for Infantile Paralysis, only to have her condition corrected through chiropractic care.

Discharged as a hopeless paraplegic in 1954, her grandparents maintained a faith beyond the polio foundation. They took their granddaughter to Dr. Lewis Robertson, a doctor of chiropractic from Glendale, California, who restored strength to her withered legs, and after six months she walked again without crutches or braces.

Mrs. Joseph Gardella, the paternal grandmother, hoping to help others who might be inflicted with this condition, signed a notarized statement complete with photographs attesting to the success with her granddaughter. Despite this, chiropractic has been and still is, totally rejected by the March of Dimes. Incredible story? Yes, indeed. But a true and thoroughly documented one.

Among entertainers who have recognized the merit of chiropractic are Enrico Caruso, Eddie Cantor, Fred Allen, Rudy Vallee, Ted Lewis, Julie Andrews, Shirley Jones, Celeste

Holm, Rock Hudson, Danny Kaye, Ryan O'Neal, Frank Sinatra, Lucille Ball, Bing Crosby, Joan Crawford, Broderick Crawford, David Janssen, Doug McClure, Robert Conrad, Robert Goulet, June Wilkinson, Arthur Godfrey, Jackie Cooper, Glenn Ford, William Holden, Mickey Rooney, June Lockhart, Inger Stevens, Don Defore, Irene Ryan, Marlo Thomas, Clint Walker, Eddie Albert, Blackstone the Magician; and Houdini, the escape artist.

Actor George Kennedy served 16 years in the military service where he received combat injuries. After back surgery and three years of braces and suffering, army doctors gave up on him. He took a medical discharge. Fortunately a friend urged that he go to a chiropractor who corrected his ailment, and he was able to begin a successful acting career.

Other well known persons who have recognized the value of chiropractic include Colonel Harland Sanders of Kentucky Fried Chicken fame; Evangelist Billy Sunday; Rev. Norman Vincent Peale; Luther Burbank, horticultural wizard; Bernarr MacFadden, editor and natural health advocate; W. Clement Stone, millionaire insurance executive; Napoleon Hill, author; Al Capp, cartoonist; Clarence Darrow, lawyer; Marcus Bach, author; Arnold Palmer and Ken Venturi, golfers; Jack Dempsey, the boxer; baseball stars Juan Marichal and Willie Mays; and Jack La Lanne, television's exercise man.

Among political leaders who have supported chiropractic are Harry S. Truman, George McGovern, Eugene McCarthy, Ronald Reagan, ~~Herbert Hoover~~, Vance Hartke, Abraham Ribicoff and Hubert Humphrey. The great lawyer and politician William Jennings Bryan subscribed to chiropractic, as did Mahatma Gandhi, the assassinated Hindu leader.

The list could go on, filling volumes with names of chiropractic friends and patients. However, it is our army of "unfamous" people that represent the most potent strength behind chiropractic. And with truth there is still more strength, strength which will assure the defeat of ignorance and propaganda.

CHAPTER XIX

A Summary

WHO CAN DENY?

CHIROPRACTIC has become the second largest healing profession in the world. In spite of medical propaganda and oppression, it continues to grow in numbers, sophistication and recognition.

Chiropractic enjoys wide recognition today, with chiropractors being licensed in 50 states, the District of Columbia and Puerto Rico. Its degree is recognized by the U.S. Office of Education, and it is classified as one of the four major healing professions by the Office of the President, Bureau of Budgets, Washington, D.C. Its colleges are accredited by the Council on Chiropractic Education approved by HEW. It is recognized by Medicare and Medicaid, by most private insurance companies, by workmen's compensation, by at least 125 congressmen who sponsored bills for chiropractic inclusion in Medicare in 1970, and by over 50 million chiropractic patients including some of the most prominent and brilliant people in the world. It also has been endorsed by numerous professional, ethnic, fraternal, veteran, senior citizen, civil service and labor organizations.

Who can deny the statistical and fact minded workmen's compensation study of thousands of patients in 44 states and Canada which, found chiropractic was "unequaled" and a "tremendous benefit" in the treatment of back conditions? Or who can deny the workmen's compensation studies, such as in the state of Florida, showing chiropractic's outstanding record of returning people back to work in 1/3 of the time and cost as compared to medicine? These are all matters of public record.

Can we deny the great contributions of the "Heretical Giants?" These courageous men and women of science advanced new concepts only to be rejected, condemned, ridiculed and persecuted by the physicians of their day, then have history recognize them years later as great heroes. As the great German poet Goethe once said, "Nothing is more endangering to a new truth than an old mistake." How tragically correct he was.

WE HAVE SEEN

We have seen organized medicine indicted for criminal action by the federal government (antitrust act), yet continue its monopolistic attitude. It has tried to eliminate the independent healing professions with resolutions, condemnations or absorption, but later copied their methods of healing. We have seen medicine teach spinal manipulation under the names of physiatry, manipulative medicine, orthopedic manipulation, rachiotherapy, orthopedic medicine, and manual medicine and at the same time, condemn chiropractic. It has tried unsuccessfully to eliminate osteopathy, first with open attack, then by absorption through kindness. It adopted resolutions condemning and prohibiting professional association with optometrists; later, while under threat of a criminal antitrust law suit, dropped all resolutions against optometry. It scoffed at podiatrists only to borrow their surgical techniques.

We have seen where organized medicine has become the largest spending lobby in American history. As every major country in the world views good health care as a "right" of its citizens, the strong influence of organized medicine has been able to keep it as a "privilege" in America.

We have seen organized medicine oppose Medicare, saying

it would violate the patients' freedom of choice of doctor. It then demonstrated gross hypocrisy by lobbying, although unsuccessfully, to keep chiropractic excluded from Medicare.

We have seen some chiropractors singled out as representative of the entire chiropractic profession, but let the profession without its sinners cast the first stone.

We have witnessed the propagandist at work, using the half-truths, innuendoes, exceptions to the rule, obsolete material, material out of context, and fallacious statements. They have been used to charge that chiropractic has no scientific evidence of its value, is against drugs, claims to have a cure-all method of healing, and is dangerous. In clarifying this confusion, we have introduced scientific and clinical proof to support the validity of chiropractic. Over 90 per cent of the chiropractors refer patients to other doctors, and this is certainly not the behavior of a profession which opposes drugs and claims to have cure-all methods of healing. The safe and ecologically sound basis of chiropractic is demonstrated by its low malpractice insurance premium rates as compared to medicine.

We have seen the chiropractic profession spend millions of dollars on its own education and research, while medical research receives millions of dollars from foundations and the federal government.

We have seen how the AMA received $18 million for research from the tobacco industry, then refused to support the surgeon general report on smoking, and opposed the Federal Trade Commission's antismoking policy, and the Federal Communication Commission's ban on cigarette advertising on radio and television. It opposed these health measures even though 95 per cent of the medical physicians believe smoking is harmful to health. We saw how the *JAMA* advertised drugs it previously condemned in previous journal articles.

We have seen that 100,000 people die and nearly 1½ million are hospitalized annually from reaction to medications. Currently, our country has one of the highest death rates of all 36 North American countries, in spite of our sophisticated and medically oriented society.

We have seen the Food and Drug Administration (FDA) investigate drugs circulated on the market, after which time 369 were found to be worthless or dangerous and were ordered off the market.

British Police blame overprescription of medications as the main cause of drug addiction in England. In our country, the drug advertising industry is contributing to drug abuse by selling escape, relief and pleasure pills. We are taught that it is more sophisticated and modern to find ease and pleasure than endure reality, disappointment and responsibility. Finally, we have found ourselves gripped in the shadows of fear for the welfare of our children and loved ones because of the drug menace which hangs so precariously over our heads, one which President Nixon characterized as "public enemy number one."

THE SUPREME LAW

Chiropractic recognizes the importance of medicine for many ailments, and when organized medicine adopts the same policy toward chiropractic it will be a great day for humanity. There is a Latin proverb: "Salus aegroti suprema lex," which means, "The welfare of the sick is the supreme law!" Chiropractic recognizes this law, when will organized medicine?

It has been said that if you repeat a lie often enough it becomes accepted as a truth. One of the world's greatest anatomists, Vesalius, was banished from his country because he disproved erroneous teachings on anatomy, teachings which went unchallenged for 1,400 years. Organized medicine's "institutionalized falsehood" of chiropractic has existed for 75 years. To perpetuate this falsehood in the light of modern evidence and understanding is to commit an inhumane and sinful act against the public.

Chiropractic, therefore, calls upon organized medicine to realize and accept the obvious truth, and abolish its prejudiced attitude toward chiropractic. It asks medicine to join hands with chiropractic, yet remain as two separate and distinct professions, working for the common good of humanity. To reject chiropractic in the light of current information is to be hopelessly blinded with prejudice. Such prejudice has no place in the healing professions.

Chiropractic must be included in state and federal research programs, in all federal health insurance programs, and its colleges must receive the same federal assistance as medical, optometric, podiatric and osteopathic schools. The patients deserve the finest in health care, and it cannot be the finest unless chiropractic is placed into proper perspective within the healing arts. In doing so, chiropractic can contribute a greater and more vital role in combatting the health crisis facing our nation. When that day comes, and it is up to all of us to do something about it now, we can truly boast of having the finest health care in the world.

WRITE YOUR CONGRESSMAN!

What can we do about this problem? Write your state and federal legislators and express your thoughts to them. They can do something about it. This is the American way. Your letter can carry influence and will speak for many.

Mailing addresses are:

(FEDERAL LEGISLATORS)

CONGRESSMAN (his name)
HOUSE OFFICE BUILDING
WASHINGTON, D.C.

SENATOR (his name)
SENATE OFFICE BUILDING
WASHINGTON, D.C.

(STATE LEGISLATORS)

HONORABLE (his name)
STATE REPRESENTATIVE
(YOUR STATE CAPITOL)

HONORABLE (his name)
STATE SENATOR
(YOUR STATE CAPITOL)

I would like to thank you for reading this book. It was written with the sincere hope of bringing light into the shadows of ignorance and prejudice in healing. Perhaps greater interprofessional understanding and tolerance will come, and with it a mutual cooperation of the healing professions in the interest of suffering humanity. If the book has served, even in part, to accomplish this goal, it was well worth the effort.

Bibliography and Notes

Bibliography and notes usually are arranged consecutively within each chapter, with notes in parenthesis.

Chapter 1. HISTORY OF MANIPULATION

Early Manipulation

Homola, Samuel, *Bonesetting, Chiropractic and Cultism,* Critique, 1963.
Dintenfass, Julius, D. C., *Chiropractic, A Modern Way to Health,* Pyramid Books, N.Y., 1970.
National Geographic, September 1971 (the manipulative experience of Capt. James Cook).

Hippocrates—Galen

Collier's Encyclopedia, P. F. Collier and Son, 1957.
Calder, Ritchie, *Medicine and Man,* New American Library, N.Y., 1962 (Hippocrates pages 63–66; Galen pages 66–71).
Garland, Joseph, M.D. *The Story of Medicine,* Houghton Mifflin Company, Boston, 1949 (Hippocrates pages 30–37; Galen pages 46–48).

The Bible

McMillen, S. I., M.D., *None of These Diseases,* Fleming H. Revell Company, Old Tappan, N.J., 1968, pages 12–13, 16.

The Dark Ages

Bryan & Bryan, *Principles and Practice of Bacteriology,* College Outline Series, Barnes & Noble, Inc., N.Y., 1951, page 5.

Haggard, Howard, M.D., *Devils Drugs and Doctors,* Harper and Brothers, 1929, Cardinal Giant Edition, 1959, pages 210–212.
Kitay, William, *The Challenge of Medicine,* Holt, Rinehart and Winston, N.Y., Chicago, San Francisco, 1963, page 21 (barber-surgeons and bloodletting).
Haggard, Howard, *Devils, Drugs, and Doctors,* Harper Brothers, 1929, Cardinal edition, pages 389–391 (the insane patient).
Homola, Samuel, *Bonesetting, Chiropractic and Cultism,* Critique, 1963 (Joseph Smith).

Chapter 2. AN INTRODUCTION TO CHIROPRACTIC

Chiropractic Origin and Growth

Palmer, D.D., *The Science, Art and Philosophy of Chiropractic,* Portland Printing House Co., 1910 (too much or not enough nerve energy; Harvey Lillard).
Bourdillon, J. F., *Spinal Manipulation,* Appleton-Century-Crofts, Meredith Corporation, London, 1970, page 131 (reference to deafness).
"Otologic Manifestations of the Cervical Syndrome," *Clinical Orthopedics,* 1962, Vol. 24, pages 34–38.

Professional Unity

Master Plan Definition, ratified by the House of Delegates in June 1964, American Chiropractic Association, Des Moines, Iowa (ACA definition).
ICA Membership Directory, International Chiropractors Association, Davenport, Iowa, 1972, page 2 (ICA definition).
Chiropractic's "White Paper" on Health, Education and Welfare Secretary's Report, *Independent Practitioners Under Medicare,* joint statement, American Chiropractic Association—International Chiropractors Association, Council of State Chiropractic Examining Boards, Inc., May 1969.

Principle and Scope of Chiropractic

Chiropractic Examining Boards and Basic Science Examining Boards, Official Directory, Council of State Chiropractic Examining Boards, 1969 (regarding licensing of chiropractic).

Adjusting Subluxations

Biedermann, Freimut, *Fundamentals of Chiropractic from the Standpoint of a Medical Doctor,* ICRC, Davenport, Iowa, 1959.

Janse, Hauser & Wells, *Chiropractic Principles and Technique*, 2nd Edition, National College of Chiropractic, Chicago, 1947.

Haldeman, S., and Drum, D., "The Compression Subluxation," *Journal of Clinical Chiropractic*, Canadian Memorial Chiropractic College, Archives Edition No. 1, Spring, 1971.

Hadley, Lee, M.D., "Intervertebral Joint Subluxation, Bony Impingement and Foramen Encroachment with Nerve Root Changes," *American Journal of Roentgenology*, Vol. 65, No. 3, March 1951.

Warbasse, James P., *Surgical Treatment*, 1937, Vol. 1, page 577.

Chiropractic and Disease

"Chiropractic the Unscientific Cult," American Medical Association, Department of Investigation, 1966 (reference to obsolete material and "single cause—single cure").

Anderson, Dewey, Ph.D., *Today's Doctor of Chiropractic*, American Chiropractic Association, Des Moines, Iowa, 1966, page 33 (an official chiropractic statement indicating that the germ theory is not denied nor is chiropractic care a cure-all).

Verner, J. Robinson, D.C., and Weiant, C.W., D.C., *The Chiropractor Looks at Infection*, A Supplement to Rational Bacteriology, New Jersey, 1942.

"The Chiropractor's Views of the Cause of Disease," *Opportunities in a Chiropractic Career*, Vocational Guidance Materials, Universal Publishing and Distribution Corporation, N.Y., 1967, page 13 (disclaiming single cause—single cure charge).

"Chiropractic," *University of Toronto Medical Journal*, February 1961 (reprint of the Canadian Chiropractic Association, Dr. Palmer stressed the diversity of cause of disease).

When to Visit a Chiropractor

Batten and Associates, Inc., Management Consultants, *Chiropractic Survey and Statistical Study*, Des Moines, Iowa, 1963 (best results experienced pages 36–37, most frequently treated pages 34–35).

Stoddard, Alan, *Manual of Osteopathic Practice*, Harper and Row, Publishers, Inc., Hoeber Medical Division, N.Y., 1969, pages 15–16.

Chapter 3. CHIROPRACTIC RECOGNITION AND VALIDITY

Chiropractic Is Recognized

Eells, Walter, Ph.D., *Academic Degrees*, U.S. Office of Education, 1960, page 169 (validity of a doctor of chiropractic degree).

Chiropractic—Its Relations with Insurance Companies, Committee on Insurance Relations, A.C.A., Des Moines, Iowa (formerly N.C.A., Webster City, Iowa, Insurances pay chiropractic claims).

A Survey and Analysis of the Treatment of Sprain and Strain Injuries in Industrial Cases, Florida Chiropractic Association Insurance Relations Committee, April 1960 (conducted by the First Research Corporation).

Gamet, I., Certified Statistical Clerk of the State of Colorado (Colorado study completed by July 21, 1950).

Barnhart, E. Paul, Consulting Actuary, *Comparison of Chiropractic Versus Medical Treatment Back Injuries,* American Chiropractic Association, 1966 (Iowa Study).

Chiropractic—*Its Relations with Insurance Companies,* American Chiropractic Association, Des Moines, Iowa (formerly NCA, Minnesota Study).

National Health Center for Health Statistics, 1963–1964, Series 10, No. 28, page 37 (4,250,000 had consulted a chiropractor from July 1963 to June 1964).

Chapter 4. CONFUSION ABOUT CHIROPRACTIC

Opinions and Reports, AMA Judicial Council, AMA Principle of Medical Ethics, 1971, Section 3, Paragraphs 7–8 (code of ethics denying MDs from referring to chiropractors).

"Physicians' Attitude Survey," *Medical Opinion,* November 1972, pages 64–65, 67 (MDs find significant value in chiropractic).

Goethe, Johanne Wolfgang Von, *Criticisms, Reflections and Maxims.*

Is Chiropractic or Medicine Scientific?

McManus, Michael W., Executive Director, Medical Society of Milwaukee County, *October 25, 1972* (letter indicating medicine is not an exact science).

"AMA Chief Urges a Chiropractic Ban," *Chicago Sun-Times,* October 24, 1969, page 34 (official AMA position is that chiropractic is an unscientific cult).

Chiropractic's Position on Drugs

Senior Citizen News, National Council of Senior Citizens, January 1969, Washington, D.C. (reprints of news by organized medicine, chiropractors discredit or ignore drug therapy).

Chiropractic Survey and Statistical Study, Batten and Associates, Inc., Management Consultants, Des Moines, Iowa, 1963, page 30, No. 74–74A (chiropractors referring patients).

Chiropractic and Vaccinations

"Why Chiropractic Cult Cannot Provide Quality Health Care," *Senior Citizens News*, National Council of Senior Citizens, Washington, D.C., 1969 (chiropractic raising doubts about smallpox).

Katz, Samuel, M.D., "Smallpox Vaccinations No Longer Advised," *Chicago Tribune*, October 23, 1971.

"Good News for Kids: Fewer Shots to Bear," *Chicago Tribune*, November 2, 1971 (American Academy of Pediatrics recommendation that smallpox vaccine no longer needed).

Van Dellen, M.D., "Smallpox Vaccine No Longer Required," *Chicago Tribune*, December 2, 1971.

"Reports Hit Safety of Some Vaccines," *Chicago Today*, November 5, 1971 (J. A. Morris, Alex Shelokov, Nicola Tauraso).

"Valueless Vaccines?" *Time Magazine*, April 17, 1972, page 68 (DBS allowing useless and dangerous vaccines to be marketed).

Chiropractic and Cancer

Chiropractic Survey and Statistical Study, Batten and Associates, Inc., Management Consultants, Des Moines, Iowa, 1963 (chiropractic and cancer, page 32, No. 77–78).

"Diagnosis Miss 26 per cent of Cancers," *Chicago Daily News*, September 27, 1972 (Boston City Hospital Study).

Chiropractors Diagnose

Chiropractic Examining Boards and Basic Science Examining Boards, Official Directory, Council of State Chiropractic Examining Boards, Cheyenne, Wyoming (subjects examined in various states and Canada).

Chiropractic "White Paper" on HEW Secretary Report *Independent Practitioners Under Medicare*, Joint ACA-ICA statement, 1969, page 9, Section III (chiropractors are trained to diagnose).

U.S. Office of Education

Academic Degrees, U.S. Office of Education, 1960 (letter from Dr. Walter Eells to General Counsel of the National Chiropractic Association—now the ACA).

Senior Citizen News, National Council of Senior Citizens, Washington, D.C., January 1969 (reference to *Academic Degrees*).

Educational Requirements of Chiropractors

Chiropractic Examining Boards and Basic Science Examining Boards, Official Directory, Cheyenne, Wyoming, 1969 (state educational requirements for chiropractors).

Educational Requirements for Licensure, Official directory of the Department of Education, American Chiropractic Association, Des Moines, Iowa, 1972.

Chiropractic "White Paper" on HEW Secretary Report *Independent Practitioners Under Medicare*, Joint ACA-ICA statement, 1969, page 7, Section I (educational requirements of chiropractors).

The Diploma Mills

Holbrook, Stewart H., *The Golden Age of Quackery*, The Macmillan Company, N.Y., 1959, pages 269–280 (reporter Harry Thompson Brundige and the *St. Louis Star*).

Smith, Ralph Lee, *At Your Own Risk*, Pocket Books, N.Y., 1969, page 10 (*Medical World News* quote of chiropractic diploma mill).

Mark, Ronnie Joan, records librarian, *Medical World News* (unpublished letter dated January 19, 1973, reference to being founded in 1960, and no record of ever making a comment of a chiropractic diploma mill).

"A New Weapon," *American Medical News*, September 15, 1969 (AMA promotion of *At Your Own Risk*).

Ran Its Course

A Survey and Analysis of Treatment of the Sprain and Strain Injuries of the Back and Neck in Industrial Cases, Florida Chiropractic Association, 1960 (study conducted by First Research Corporation).

It's All in Your Mind

Ussher, Neville, "The Viscerospinal Syndrome," *Annals of Internal Medicine*, Vol. 13, No. 11 (spinal manipulation for visceral disorders).

Chiropractic Proven Safe

Parsons, W.B., M.D., "Vertebral Manipulations," *Journal of the College of General Practice of Canada*, July 1965 (reference to propaganda against the safety of spinal manipulation as unfounded and false).

United States Fidelity and Guaranty Co., Chicago, Ill. (letter dated September 21, 1971 from Robert Jasker, casualty department—malpractice rates).

Insurance Services Offices suggested rates (Los Angeles effective July 5, 1972; New York effective October 4, 1972).

"Malpractice Suits Rise, Lead Doctors to Treat Patients with Caution," *Wall Street Journal*, January 8, 1971, page 1.

Wunsch, Leo, II, D.C., National Chiropractic Insurance Company, Des Moines, Iowa, December 27, 1972 (letter to its policyholders indicating no increase in rates since NCIC was organized in 1946).

Chiropractic and Medical Malpractice

Smith, Ralph Lee, *At Your Own Risk*, Pocket Books, N.Y., 1969, prologue (California case of cancer of the eye).

Haynes, George, D.C., *Chirogram*, August 1970 (a study of medical malpractice and law violations).

"Ralph Nader Reports," *Ladies Home Journal*, September 1972 (comments by Eli Burnsweig and Abe Ribicoff).

"Malpractice Suits Raise Doctors' Fears," *Chicago Today*, December 12, 1971, page 8 (President Nixon's commission on malpractice).

"Nader Aide Says 10,000 Die Yearly in Needless Surgery," *Chicago Tribune*, December 17, 1971 (study by Sidney Wolfe).

Kramer, Charles, *The Negligent Doctor*, Crown Publishing, Inc., N.Y., 1968.

Gross, Martin, *The Doctors*, Random House, N.Y., 1966, page 515 (Attorney Kramer comments on malpractice ratio to malpractice suits).

"Physician, Heal Thyself," *Chicago Sun-Times*, April 4, 1971, page 34 (Sen. Abraham Ribicoff's subcommittee report).

Lewis, Howard and Martha, *The Medical Offenders*, Simon and Schuster, N.Y., 1970, page 21.

Derbyshire, Robert C., "What Should the Profession Do About the Incompetent Physician?" *JAMA*, December 20, 1965.

Hoffman, Daniel, *Rocky Mountain News*, September 24, 1970 (inadequate internal policing in Colorado).

Lack of Referral—A Potential Danger

Haldeman, S., and Meyer B. J., "The Effect of Experimental Construction on the Structure of The Sciatic Nerve," *South African Journal of Laboratory and Clinical Medicine*, August 8, 1970, pages 888–892.

Haldeman S. and Meyer B. J., "The Effect of Construction on the Conduction of The Action Potential in the Sciatic Nerve," *South African Journal of Laboratory and Clinical Medicine*, August 8, 1970, pages 903–906.

Bourdillon, J. F., *Spinal Manipulation*, Appleton-Century-Crofts, Educational Division, Meredith Corporation, London, 1970, page 132 (reference to 15 years in practice and trophic changes noted).

Schimmel, Elihu, *Annals of Internal Medicine*, January 1964, pages 100–110 (a national projection of the Yale-New Haven Study of iatrogenic episodes).

"Senseless Surgery—Are 3,000,000 Operations Each Year Unnecessary?" *The National Observer*, July 29, 1972 (one in five operations unnecessary).

The Tardiness of Louisiana

Adams, Paul, D.C., *ACA Journal of Chiropractic*, January 1970, page 23 (United States Supreme Court and the England Case).

Nineteenth Judicial District Court, East Baton Rouge Parish, State of Louisiana, Civil Docket No. 73, 676, Jerry R. England, et. al. Plaintiffs versus Louisiana State Board of Medical Examiners, et. al., Defendants (plaintiffs' original memorandum, council for plaintiffs J. Minos Simon and Floyd J. Reed of Louisiana, Russel Morton Brown of Washington, D.C.).

United States District Court, Eastern District of Louisiana, New Orleans Division, Civil Action No. 9, 292, Jerry England, et. al., Plaintiffs versus Louisiana Board of Medical Examiners, et. al., Defendants (original brief of plaintiffs)..

"Chiropractic: The Unscientific Cult," American Medical Association, Department of Investigation, 1966, page 22 (material out of context, "since chiropractic claims to be a complete and independent art").

"Statement of Policy on Chiropractic Adopted by AMA House of Delagates," *JAMA*, November 1966, April 17, 1967. Vol. 200, No. 3 (using material out of context "since chiropractic claims to be a complete and independent art").

Wisconsin Task Force Report

Report of the Chiropractic Study Committee to The Governor's Health Planning and Policy Task Force, Madison, Wisconsin, October 23, 1972 (total pages 41).

Milwaukee Journal, October 28, 1972 (a letter to David Carly, Task Force Chairman, from Dr. David J. Carlson commenting on task force report).

Milwaukee Sentinel, October 28, 1972 (same as *Milwaukee Journal* above).

(The National College of Chiropractic in Lombard, Ill., was passed enroute to the Palmer College of Chiropractic in Davenport, Iowa).

Chiropractic's "White Paper" on HEW Secretary Report, *Independent Practitioners Under Medicare*, May 1969 (provided rebuttal).

Back Injuries, A Major Health Problem in the United States, Department of Research and Statistics, American Chiropractic Association, 1966 (reports of workmen's compensation by states).

"Must Unify Health Care, Lucey says," *Milwaukee Journal*, March 28, 1973 (Wisconsin Task Force Report by governor excludes reference to chiropractic).

Chapter 5. TOOLS OF THE PROPAGANDISTS

Holmes, Oliver Wendell, M.D., *The Autocrat of the Breakfast Table.*

Hitler, Adolf, *Mein Kampf*, British Foreign Policy Association translation, 1935 (written in prison 1923 with the aid of Hess and Rauschning).

Smith, Ralph Lee, "Visit to a Bizarre World—Chiropractic Alma Maters," *Today's Health*, July 1968 (AMA publication using various tools, half-truths, innuendoes, material out of context, etc.).

Smith, Ralph Lee, *At Your Own Risk*, Pocket Books, N.Y. 1969 (promoted by AMA using the above "tools").

"Why Chiropractic Cult Cannot Provide Quality Health Care," *Senior Citizen News*, National Council of Senior Citizens, Washington, D.C., January 1969 (classic 2 page summary of "tools" of propagandists as reprinted and circulated by the AMA).

Landers, Ann, *Chicago Sun Times*, January 28, 1971 (innuendo licensed by medical board of examiners).

Chiropractic: The Unscientific Cult, Official AMA publication, Department of Investigation, Chicago, Illinois, 1966.

What They Say About Chiropractic, Official AMA publication, Chicago, Illinois (typical tools of propagandist).

Maisel, Albert Q., "Should Chiropractors Be Paid With Your Tax Dollars?" *Readers Digest*, July 1971, pages 76–81 (typical propaganda article as supported by the AMA).

Innuendoes

Gearhart, Louis, Director of Professional Affairs, *Coverage of Chiropractic Services in Workmen's Compensation Insurance*, Des Moines, Iowa. March 1, 1968.

"Chiropractic Mounts Major Political Drive," *American Medical News*, January 24, 1972, pages 10–11 (statement that New Mexico and Connecticut dropped chiropractic in Medicaid).

State of Connecticut, State Welfare Department, Hartford, unpublished letter dated March 13, 1972 (James F. Morrison, Director of Health Administration, stating chiropractic is *not* cancelled in Connecticut, refuting January 24, 1972 AMA statement).

Obsolete Material

Smith, Ralph Lee, *At Your Own Risk*, Pocket Books, N.Y., 1969 (false reference to 22 states requiring chiropractic to have 1 or 2 years college).

Chiropractic Examining Boards and Basic Science Examining Boards Official Directory, Council of State Chiropractic Examining Boards, Cheyenne, Wyoming, 1969 (confirmation of state requirements to practice chiropractic).

Material Out of Context and Half-Truths

Smith, Ralph Lee, *At Your Own Risk*, Pocket Books, N.Y., 1969, page 41 (reference to being in love).

Garland, Joseph, M.D., *The Story of Medicine*, Houghton Mifflin Company, Boston, 1949, pages 33, 86 (reference to Hippocrates and love).

Gross, Martin, *The Doctors*, Random House, N.Y., 1966, pages 354–355 (the doctor as a businessman).

Chapter 6. CHIROPRACTIC IN MEDICARE

HEW Report

Cohen, Wilbur J., *Independent Practitioners Under Medicare*, Department of Health, Education and Welfare, December 28, 1968 (Ad Hoc consultant group list on pages 212–214; Expert Review Panel on page 215).

Independent Practitioners Under Medicare, joint statement, American Chiropractic Association—International Chiropractors Association, Council of State Chiropractic Examining Boards, Inc., May 1969 (chiropractic's "White Paper" on Health, Education and Welfare Secretary's Report).

The HEW Octopus

Journal of the American Medical Association, September 15, 1969 (reference to "unbiased" HEW report).

Sabatier, Joseph A., M.D., *"At Your Own Risk: The Case Against Chiropractic," JAMA*, September 15, 1969, Vol. 209, No. 11 (AMA editorial making reference to HEW's "unbiased study" on chiropractic).

Kennedy, Edward, *Congressional Record*, Senate, October 5, 1972, Vol. 118, No. 159 (recommending a chiropractic study).

Chiropractic Cost Study in Medicine

Barnhart, E. Paul, consulting actuary, American Chiropractic Association, Des Moines, Iowa (testimony before the House Ways and Means Committee, November 3, 1969, regarding SSA false 26 per cent increase, 19 insurance companies).

Higley, Henry, M.A., D.C., *Back Injuries—A Major Health Problem in the United States*, Department of Research and Statistics, Committee on Insurance Industrial and Labor Relations, American Chiropractic Association, Des Moines, Iowa, 1966.

Barnhart, E. Paul, Consulting Actuary, *Comparison of Chiropractic verses Medical Treatment Back Injuries*, American Chiropractic Association, 1966 (Iowa Study).

Gamet, I., Certified Statistical Clerk of the State of Colorado, study completed July 21, 1950.

Chiropractic—Its Relations with Insurance Companies, American Chiropractic Association, Des Moines, Iowa (formerly NCA—Minnesota study).

"Comparative Cost Studies," American Chiropractic Association, Des Moines, Iowa, 1971 (cost studies from statistical information furnished by Oregon workmen's compensation board).

"Kansas Workmen's Compensation Study," American Chiropractic Association, Des Moines, Iowa, 1971.

Higley, Henry, D.C., "Chiropractic in Public Assistance Medical Care in the State of California," *The Chirogram*, March 1968, Vol. 35, No. 3.

Labor and Chiropractic, American Chiropractic Association, Des Moines, Iowa.

A Survey and Analysis of Treatment of the Sprain and Strain of Injuries of the Back and Neck in Industrial Cases, Florida Chiropractic Association, 1960 (study conducted by the First Research Corporation).

Back Injuries—A Major Health Problem in the United States Department of Research and Statistics of the American Chiropractic Association, 1966, page 7 (one billion dollar cost).

Freedom of Choice of Health Care

"Why Chiropractic Cult Cannot Provide Quality Health Care," *Senior Citizen News*, National Council of Senior Citizens, Washington, D.C., January 1969 (reference to chiropractic's political drive).

Harris, Richard, *A Sacred Trust*, Penguin Books, Inc., 1969, pages 123–125 (AMA opposition to national health care).

Cook, Fred J., *The Plot Against the Patient*, Prentice-Hall, Inc., Englewood Cliffs, N.J., 1967 (Sir Luke Fildes' painting).

Annis, Edward, "Political Action Conference," *Human Events Newsletter*, 1963 (Medicare is a hoax and a fraud).

Joint Statement of ACA and ICA before Republican Task Force on National Health Care, Washington, D.C., May 31, 1972, page 4 (insurance equality laws).

Chapter 7. MEDICINE'S OPPOSITION TO MEDICARE

"A Call to Arms," *Journal of the American Medical Association*, August 16, 1971, Vol. 217, No. 7 (AMA's lobbying to exclude chiropractic from Medicare).

Harris, Richard, *A Sacred Trust*, Penguin Books, Inc., 1969, pages 128–129 (Professor William Demougeot addressing the AMA officers in Chicago).

Health Crisis

Kennedy, Edward, *In Critical Condition—The Crisis in America's Health Care*, Simon and Schuster, 1972, pages 15–16.

Better Spending Needed

Ehrenreich, Barbara and Richard, *"The American Health Empire,"* Vintage Books, N.Y., 1971, pages 147–163.

De Vise, Pierre, *Journal American Hospital Association*, February 1, 1971 (the five points, page 53; teletherapy units, page 54; exhorbitant health care, page 55).

From Crisis Therapy to Health Care, A Study in the Development of Alternatives, Student Research Facility, Berkeley, California, 1972, page 5 ($80 billion for health care in 1971).

Organized Medicine's Real Reason For Opposing Medicare

"U.S. Refuses 'High' Medicare Payments," *Chicago Tribune*, April 13, 1972.

"Excess Doctor Fees Set at $500 Million" *Chicago Tribune*, March 1, 1972.

Chapter 8. THE NATIONAL COUNCIL OF SENIOR CITIZENS

"Why Chiropractic Cult Cannot Provide Quality Health Care," *Senior Citizen News*, National Council of Senior Citizens, Washington, D.C., 1969.

Polish-American Senior Citizens

Kiel, Eleanor Deka, director of the National and Chicago Area Councils of Senior Citizen and Vice President of Polish-American Senior Citizens, unpublished letter dated November 29, 1969 (statement refuting the *Senior Citizen News* article on chiropractic).

Nordheimer, Roy, President, Chicago Area Council of Senior Citizen Organizations, Chicago, Ill., December 16, 1969 (letter concurring with Mrs. Kiel's letter).

Schroedter, Ed, President, Allied Councils of Senior Citizens of Wisconsin, Inc., Milwaukee, Wisconsin (letter dated December 28, 1969 concurring with Mrs. Kiel's letter).

Chapter 9. CHIROPRACTIC AND THE AMA

"AMA Chief Urges a Chiropractic Ban," *Chicago Sun-Times*, October 24, 1969 (monopoly).

"Chiropractors as Physician's Assistants?" *Medical Economic News*, April 12, 1971, page 48.

"Ex-Chiropractors Enter Training as MD's Assistants," *American Medical News*, November 15, 1971, pages 8–9.

"A New Weapon," *American Medical News*, September 15, 1969 (AMA's promotion of Smith's book).

Smith, Ralph Lee, "I Was Awarded a Chiropractor Certificate After a 3-Day Course," *National Enquirer*, January 1969.

Potterton, Reginald, "I Cut Out Her Heart and Stomped on it!" Playboy Magazine, April 1969 (discussing the *National Enquirer*).

Antitrust Act Violated

Harris, Richard, *A Sacred Trust*, Penguin Books, Inc. 1969. Page 17 (federal employees for Group Health Association).

Organized Medicine's Questionable Behavior

Harris, Richard, *A Sacred Trust*, Penguin Books, Inc., 1969 (AMPAC formed, page 134–136; United Steelworkers, page 155).

Summers, John, M.D., "AMA and Tobacco," *Medical Tribune*, November 30, 1970 (AMA and its tobacco-subsidized committee).

Harris, Richard, *A Sacred Trust*, Penguin Books, Inc., 1969, pages 159–161 (AMA and the tobacco industry).

Medical World News, April 10, 1964 (AMA's opposition to FTC ruling on cigarettes).

Medical Tribune, April 3, 1964 (AMA's opposition to FTC ruling on cigarettes).

Medical Tribune, July 4, 1968 (AMA's "complex" study on smoking to be done "slowly").

Medical Tribune, February 17, 1969 (AMA opposition to FCC ruling on cigarette advertising).

American Medical News, March 16, 1970 (ban on television advertising of cigarettes, also deadline for warning on package of cigarettes).

Summers, John E., M.D., "Conflict of Interest," *Medical Tribune*, April 5, 1972 (AMA lack of initiative with tobacco and addictive drugs).

Food and Drug Administration, Bureau of Drugs, National Academy of Sciences—National Research Council Drug Efficacy Study Group, November 1, 1970 (369 drugs condemned and ordered off market).

"Fixed Combinations of Antimicrobial Agents," *New England Journal of*

Medicine, National Academy of Science—National Research Council Division of Medical Sciences Drug Efficacy Study, Vol. 280, No. 21, May 22, 1969.

Wilkins, Lawson, M.D., *Journal of the American Medical Association*, Vol. 172, No. 10, March 5, 1960 (masculinized baby girls).

Medical Dissention

"Mississippi Makes AMA Dues Voluntary," *American Medical News*, May 24, 1971 (Mississippi and Nebraska societies vote against compulsory AMA memberships).

"AMA Orders Cuts to Trim Losses, Streamline Group," *Chicago-Tribune*, October 26, 1972.

"AMA Ranks Thin as Leaders Split on Goals," *Chicago-Tribune*, December 13, 1971, pages 1–2 (allowing interns and residents to join AMA).

"Medical Students Win AMA Policy Vote," *Chicago Daily News*, December 1, 1971.

"What Doctors Think of Their Patients," *Life Magazine*, October 2, 1970, pages 68–72 (Harris Poll).

"Young Doctors Snubbing AMA," *Chicago Today*, September 5, 1971, page 54 (Committee for Human Rights).

"Young Doctor Snubbing AMA," *Chicago Today*, September 5, 1971, page 54 (New York dropped AMA mandatory membership; reference to National Staff Conference; Ernest B. Howard, turmoil in the organization).

Lynfield, Joshua, M.D., *American Medical News*, December 21, 1970 (AMA claims to represent medicine without knowing its views).

Medicine's Political Drive

"Chiropractic Mounts Major Political Drive," *American Medical News*, January 24, 1972 (emphasis on chiropractics' political drive).

"The Nation's Worst Scandal," *Chicago Sun-Times*, Parade Section, March 21, 1971, page 5 (AMPAC's $700,000 in contributions).

"1965 Lobby Spending Was Highest in 14 Years," *Congressional Record Almanac*, 1966.

"AMA Group Blocked Me, Knowles says," *Chicago Tribune*, June 28, 1969 (AMA's rejection of Knowles).

"Dr. Knowles to Head Rockefeller Foundation," *Chicago Sun-Times*, September 14, 1971, page 23 (AMA's rejection of Knowles).

"Ted Fires New Salvo at AMA," *Chicago Daily News*, July 15, 1971, page 28 (Washington UPI statement of Edward Kennedy's attack on AMA).

"Teddy Calls AMA Note 'Blackmail'," *Chicago Tribune*, July 23, 1971, Section 1-A, page 3.

Dintenfass, Julius, D.C., "Bill to Abolish Chiropractic Defeated at 1971 Model Congress," *The ACA Journal of Chiropractic*, May 1971, page 44.
Harris, Richard, *A Sacred Trust*, Penguin Books, Inc., 1969 (the political drives and questionable dealings of organized medicine).

Chiropractic's Political Drive

McAndrews, J. F., D.C., executive director of the International Chiropractors Association, Davenport, Iowa, September 22, 1971 (unpublished letter regarding legislative costs).
"The American Chiropractic Association and You!" The American Chiropractic Association, Des Moines, Iowa, 1972, page 2 (40 per cent dues for education and research).
Foundation for Chiropractic Education and Research, Ames, Iowa, 1972, page 1 (40% ACA funds for education and research).
Autopsy on the AMA, Student Research Facility, Berkeley, California, 1971 (AMA record of opposition to reform).
Harris, Richard, *A Sacred Trust*, Penguin Books, Inc., 1969 (AMA record of opposition to reform).

Money Cannot Buy

"Public Demand for Chiropractic," Joint Statement of the American Chiropractic Association and International Chiropractors Association before Republican Task Force on National Health, U.S. House of Representatives, Washington D.C., May 31, 1972, page 2 (regarding majority of AFL-CIO membership and the Chamber of Commerce of the United States).
"Unified Chiropractic Statement on Inclusion of Chiropractic Services in Medicare," Joint ACA-ICA statement, November 3, 1969 (chiropractic testimony before Congress on Medicare).

The Doctor Shortage and the AMA

"The People Left Behind," President's National Advisory Commission on Rural Poverty, September 1967, pages 59, 63.
Gerber, Alex, M.D., *The Gerber Report*, David McKay Company, Inc., N.Y., 1971 (5,000 communities, pages 44–45; Magnuson and Bane Commission, page 48; Russians exporting MDs, page 57).
"An Army of 600,000 Doctors," *USSR Health Service*, USSR publication, 1970, page 13.
Gross, Martin, *The Doctors*, Random House, N.Y., 1966 (shortage of doctors and the AMA pages 478–79.
"What the Doctors Ordered?" *Chicago Sun Times*, August 27, 1971 (1,000 persons die in Chicago annually according to Pierre de Vise).

Chapter 10. CHIROPRACTIC AND MEDICAL EDUCATION

Flexner, Abraham, *Medical Education in the United States and Canada*, Carnegie Foundation, N.Y., 1910 (31 of the existing 155 schools deserved to exist, page 28; plague spot of the country, page 216; California Medical College, Oakland, page 190; San Francisco Hahnemann school "the instructor doesn't believe in it," page 159; the five eclectic schools, page 162; six schools remain all utterly hopeless, page 160; European trip, page 19, footnotes; exaggerations, misstatements, page 19; one utterly wretched room, page 19, footnotes; ignorant and clumsy, pages 36–37; dirty pigeonhole, no protection against fraud or forgery, page 36; go a long way on faith, nonexistent schools, nonexistent places, page 36; course less than 6 months, page 11).

Gross, Martin, *The Doctors*, Random House, N.Y., 1966, pages 397–398 (5 school study of grade averages).

"Medical Education in the United States," *Journal of the American Medical Association*, November 25, 1968, Vol. 206, No. 9, page 2014.

Chiropractic Education

Saunders Report, International Chiropractors Association, Davenport, Iowa, 1958.

"Some Comments on the Educational Standards and Standing of Colleges of Chiropractic," *Badger Report*, National Council on Education of the National Chiropractic Association, Des Moines, Iowa, 1960 (Council on Chiropractic Education).

"Chiropractic Survey and Statistical Study," Batten and Associates Inc., Management Consultants, Des Moines, Iowa, 1963, page 36, No. 81 (poll of standard of chiropractic education for accreditation).

"Educational Standards for Chiropractic Colleges," Council on Chiropractic Education, Des Moines, Iowa, Ninth Revision, 1970, pages 1–20 (accreditation and standards for chiropractic colleges).

"Criteria and Procedures for Evaluation of Chiropractic Colleges," Association of Chiropractic Colleges, pages 1–34 (objectives, criterion and guidelines for evaluation).

National State Presidents' Congress, Washington, D.C., 1970 (resolution for two year college prerequisite for entrance into chiropractic college).

U.S. Office of Education

Gerber, Alex, M.D., *The Gerber Report*, David McKay Company, Inc., N.Y., 1971, page 61 (cost of building a medical school).

Chapter 11. HERETICAL GIANTS

Garland, Joseph, M.D., *The Story of Medicine*, Houghton Mifflin Company, Boston, 1949 (general reference).
Calder, Ritchie, *Medicine and Man*, New American Library, N.Y., 1962, pages 90–91.
Haggard, Howard, *The Doctor in History*, Yale University Press, Oxford, Connecticut, 1934 (general reference).

Paracelsus

Haggard, Howard, M.D., *Devils, Drugs and Doctors*, Harper and Brothers, 1929, Cardinal Giant edition, Chapter 15, pages 362–66 (Paracelsus).
Garland, Joseph, M.D., *The Story of Medicine*, Houghton Mifflin Company, Boston, 1949, page 71.
Poole, Lynn and Gray, *Doctors Who Saved Lives*, Dodd, Mead and Company, N.Y., 1966, page 19 (Paracelsus using tissue manipulation on Frobenius).

Michael Servetus

Haggard, Howard, *The Doctor in History*, Yale University Press, New Haven, Connecticut, 1934, pages 244–245.
Haggard, Howard, M.D., *Devils, Drugs and Doctors*, Harper and Brothers, 1929, Cardinal Giant Edition, Chapter 6, page 153 (Servetus).

Andreas Vesalius

Haggard, Howard, M.D., *Devils, Drugs and Doctors*, Harper and Brothers, 1929, Cardinal Giant Edition, pages 149–155 (Andreas Vesalius).
Garland, Joseph, M.D., *The Story of Medicine*, Houghton Mifflin Company, Boston, 1949, pages 73–75.
Shippen, Katherine B., *Men of Medicine*, Viking Press, N.Y., 1957, pages 82–83.
Hume, Ruth Fox, *Great Men of Medicine*, Random House, N.Y., 1961.

William Harvey

One Hundred Great Lives, Edited by John Allen, Greystone Press, N.Y., 1948.
Shippen, Katherine B., *Men of Medicine*, Viking Press, N.Y., 1957, pages 91–93.

George Bodington

Solomon, Saul, M.D., *Tuberculosis*, Coward-McCann, Inc., N.Y., 1952.

Ignaz Semmelweis

McMillen, S. I., M.D., *None of These Diseases*, Fleming H. Revell Company, Old Tappan, N.J., 1968, pages 13–15.
Haggard, Howard, M.D., *Devils, Drugs & Doctors*, Harper and Brothers, 1929, Cardinal Giant Edition, Chapter 4, pages 85–93.
Thompson, Morton, *The Cry and the Covenant*, Signet Books, 1969.

Louis Pasteur

Haggard, Howard W., M.D., *Devils, Drugs and Doctors*, Harper and Brothers, 1929, pages 377–378.
Hume, Ruth Fox, *Great Men of Medicine*, Random House, N.Y., 1961.
Shippen, Katherine B., *Men of Medicine*, Viking Press, N.Y., 1957, pages 119–120.

Joseph Lister

One Hundred Great Lives, Edited by John Allen, Graystone Press, N.Y., 1948, pages 640–647.
Hume, Ruth Fox, *Great Men of Medicine*, Random House, N.Y., 1961, pages 115–116.

Florence Nightingale

Dodge, Bertha S., *The Story of Nursing*, Little, Brown and Company, Boston, 1965, pages 15–37.
McKown, Robin, *Heroic Nurses*, G. P. Putnam's Sons, N.Y., 1966, pages 51–71.
Haggard, Howard, M.D., *Devils, Drugs and Doctors*, Harper and Brothers, 1929, Cardinal Giant Edition, pages 175–176.

Sister Elizabeth Kenny

McKown, Robin, *Heroic Nurses*, G. P. Putnam's Sons, N.Y., 1966, pages 189–211.

Lorraine M. Golden

"Program Restores Hope," *The ACA Journal of Chiropractic*, April 1971 (reprint of *The Louisville Cardinal*, October 2, 1970).
Smith, Jerome, "The Kentuckiana Story," Kentuckiana Center for Education, Health and Research, Inc., Louisville, Kentucky, May 1970.
"Center for Handicapped Is Attacked and Defended," *The Courier—Journal and Times*, July 30, 1967.

The Insight of Kentuckiana, Official publication of Kentuckiana Center for Health, Education and Research, November 1970, November 1971, February 1972.

Leo L. Spears

"Spears Hospital—The Dream That Came True," *Spears Sanigram*, Denver, Colorado, June–July 1971.

Chapter 12. DANIEL DAVID PALMER

Ingersoll, Robert G., *Liberty of Man, Woman and Child.*

Self Educated

Flexner, Abraham, *Medical Education in the United States and Canada*, Carnegie Foundation, N.Y., 1910, page 28 (155 medical schools, all but 31 diploma mills).

Kane, Joseph, *Facts About the Presidents*, Permabooks, N.Y., 1960 (facts on Lincoln, Truman).

One Hundred Great Lives, Edited by John Allen, Greystone Press, N.Y., 1948 (Florence Nightingale).

Halgrim, Robert C., *The Edison Record*, Ft. Meyers, Florida, undated, page 29 (1,097 patents).

Poole, Lynn and Gray, *Men Who Pioneered Inventions*, Dodd, Mead and Company, N.Y., 1969, pages 32–45 (shop keeper and wine gauger).

Garland, Joseph, M.D., *The Story of Medicine*, Houghton Mifflin Company, Boston, 1949, pages 102–103 (Leeuwenhoek developing the microscope).

Palmer, D. D., *The Science, Art and Philosophy of Chiropractic*, Portland Printing House Company, 1910.

Chapter 13. MEDICAL PLAGIARISM, MONOPOLY AND BIGOTRY

Chiropractic

Savage, L. J., D.C., "Call for Peace Among Healing Professions," *Journal of the California Chiropractic Association*, April 1971 (Dr. Savage addressing University of California symposium).

Podiatry

Podell, Richard N., M.D., "Issues in the Organization of Medical Care," *New England Journal of Medicine*, March 18, 1971, pages 586–589.

Optometry

Bass, Cyrus, O.D., "Report to the Optometric Profession," Principal plaintiff in relation to Dr. Cyrus Bass, et al., vs. The American Medical Association, et al., in the U.S. District Court for the Northern District of Illinois, Eastern Division (23 pages, and exhibits A through F).
"Houston Optometrists Sue Ophthalmological Society," *American Medical News*, August 9, 1971.

Osteopathy

AOA-AMA Relationship, American Osteopathic Association, Chicago, Illinois, *White Paper*, No. 1, May 1965; *White Paper*, No. 2, March 1968; *White Paper*, No. 3, August 1970.

Conclusion

King, David, U.S. Representative, 89th Congress, Washington, D.C. (question asked publicly).

Chapter 14. HEALTH ABUSE

United Nations Population and Vital Statistics

Population and Vital Statistics Report, Statistical Papers, Department of Economic and Social Affairs, Series A, Vol. 22, No. 3, United Nations, N.Y., July 1, 1970, pages 11–15.

Nutrition Abuse

"Starvation on 'Enriched' Bread," *Des Moines Register*, October 22, 1970 (reprinted in *Healthway Magazine*, February 1971, page 17).
"Research on Obesity," *Healthways Magazine*, American Chiropractic Association, Des Moines, Iowa, May 1971, page 20 (Dr. Rimm).
"Obesity," *Merck Manual*, Merck and Company, Inc., Rahway, N.J., 1966, 11th Edition, page 324 (death rate with overweight).
Cook, James, *Remedies and Rackets*, W. W. Norton and Company, Inc., N.Y. 1958, pages 106–107 (reducing pills).

Medication Abuse

Larrick, George P., "Beware: The New Medical Quacks," *Parade*, December 18, 1955 ("good old days").
Cook, James, *Remedies and Rackets*, W. W. Norton and Company, Inc., N.Y. 1958 (little protection against ineffective drugs and deceptive advertising).

Kreig, Margaret, *Black Market Medicine*, Prentice Hall, Inc., Inglewood Cliffs, N.J., page 91 (pharmacists production managers discussion).
"Nixon Gets Osteopathic Treatment Twice a Month," *Chicago Sun-Times*, April 11, 1972 (W. Kenneth Riland, D.O.).
ACA-ICA Statement before Republican Task Force on National Health, Washington, D.C., May 31, 1972, page 2 (health system not a sickness system).
"Medics Biggest Drug Menace," *D. C. Digest*, National Springwall Associates, Brighton, Colorado, Digest No. 15 (13 billion barbiturates).
"Drug Dependent Society," *Healthways Magazine*, American Chiropractic Association, Des Moines, Iowa, May 1970, page 5 (22,000 drug products, 10 million pounds of aspirin).

Deep Concern

Reimann, Hobart, M.D., *Healthways Magazine*, American Chiropractic Association, January 1971, pages 26–27 (quoting *N.Y. Times*, April 19, 1966).
Boyd, William, M.D., *A Textbook of Pathology, An Introduction to Medicine*, Lea and Febiger, Philadelphia, 1961.
Moser, Robert H., M.D., *Diseases of Medical Progress*, Charles C. Thomas, Ft. Lauderdale, Florida, 1969.
Spain, David M., M.D., *The Complications of Modern Medical Practice*, Grune and Stratton, N.Y., 1963 (iatrogenic disease).
"Aspirin Can Cause Death, Doctor Warns," *Chicago Tribune*, October 13, 1970 (Rene Menguy).
"Dangers of Aspirin Cited," *Healthways Magazine*, American Chiropractic Association, Des Moines, Iowa, October 1971, page 11 (Rodale's Health Bulletin—Dr. Naiman and aspirin).
"Doctor Deplores Drug Use for Colds," *Healthways Magazine*, American Chiropractic Association, Des Moines, Iowa, October, 1971 (Dr. Paul Stolley).
Mintz, Morton, *The Therapeutic Nightmare*, Houghton Mifflin Company, Boston, 1965.
Chicago Daily News, November 4, 1971 (comments by Senator Gaylord Nelson on misrepresenting, distorting and withholding information).
Johnson, George, *The Pill Conspiracy*, New American Library, N.Y., 1967, pages 16–17 (Hubert Humphrey).
Food and Drug Administration, Bureau of Drugs, National Academy of Sciences—National Research Council Drug Efficacy Study Group, November 1, 1970.
"Deemed Ineffective or Dangerous—FDA Blacklist of Drug Products," *Chicago Today*, November 29, 1970, page 26.

"Study Reveals Mislabeling in Drug Industry," *Chicago Tribune*, November 29, 1970, Section 1A, page 14 (Dr. Robert Cannan).

The Fond Du Lac Study, The American Medical Association, Chicago, 1955.

"The Over-Medicated Woman," *McCall's Magazine*, September 1971, page 67 ($800 million a year promoting medical products in medical journals).

Schimmel, Elihu, M.D., "The Hazards of Hospitalization," *Annals of Internal Medicine*, January 1964, pages 100–110 (Yale-New Haven study of iatrogenic reactions).

Spain, David, M.D., *The Complications of Modern Medical Practices*, Grune and Stratton, N.Y., 1963.

Cluff, Leighton, M.D., "Are Drug Effects Controllable?" *Medical World News*, June 18, 1965, page 40.

Drug Addiction

"Still Dying for a Smoke?" *Reader's Digest*, July 1971, pages 49–52.

Lasagna, Louis, M.D., *Life, Death and the Doctor*, Alfred A. Knopf, N.Y., 1968 (smoking, emphysema and cancer).

Smoking and Health, U.S. Department of HEW, Publication No. 1103, 1964, pages 300–302 (summary on emphysema, bronchitis and pregnancy, premature deliveries defined as 2,500 grams or less).

"Smoking and Heart Disease," American Heart Association, N.Y., 1964 (death rate 50–200 per cent higher among smokers).

"Tobacco Trade Aid Draws Fire," *Chicago Daily News*, July 14, 1971, page 43 (Senator Frank Moss).

Mintz, Morton, *The Therapeutic Nightmare*, Houghton Mifflin Company, Boston, 1965 (pharmaceutical industry supporting AMA).

"Why Young People Turn to Drugs," *Reader's Digest*, September 1972, pages 106–110.

Hollister, William, M.D., "Combating the Drug Peril," *PTA Magazine*, March 1971, pages 2–5.

"What Our Children Say About Drugs," *Chicago Today*, April 19, 1971, pages 25–26 (smoking pot, T.V. commercials, excerpts from the book *"You, Your Child and Drugs,"* by the Child Study Association of America).

"Drug Overdose Deaths Spiraling: Dr. Toman," *Park Ridge Herald*, May 13, 1971, page 33 (drug overdose deaths).

"Drug Overdose Deaths Hit Alltime High," *Pickwick Newspapers*, January 20, 1972 (drug overdose deaths).

"Drug Deaths Here up 22 per cent," *Chicago Tribune*, April 15, 1972 (drug overdose deaths).

"The Status of Discipline in the Medical Profession," *Federation Bulletin*, January 1960.

"British Punish for 'Overprescribing'," *Healthways Magazine*, American Chiropractic Association, Des Moines, Iowa, October 1970, page 41.

Conclusion

Haynes, George H., D.C., *Analysis and Evaluation of Chiropractic Education in the United States*, Glendale, California, May 1960 (survey comparing 11 chiropractic and 77 medical colleges courses in nutrition).
Slee, V.N., M.D., "Streamlining the Tissue Committee," *Bulletin, American College of Surgeons*, November–December 1959, page 519 (survey of mastectomy, gastrectomy, appendectomy, uterus operations, gall bladder surgery, operation on tubes and/or ovaries, and operations on the thyroid).
"Tonsillectomy and Adenoidectomy," *Canadian Medical Association Journal*, December 28, 1963, pages 1334–1335 (statistics on death from tonsillectomy, and Dr. W. J. E. McKee study).
Sparling, Dr. J. Frederick, from Johns Hopkins studied 1002 appendectomies in 5 hospitals which showed less than one-half were necessary.
"Hysterectomy Trends," *The Record*, Commission on Professional and Hospital Activities, March 25, 1965.
Doyle, James, M.D., "Unnecessary Hysterectomies," *JAMA*, January 31, 1953, pages 360–365 (study of 6,248 operations in thirty hospitals during 1948).

Chapter 15. CHIROPRACTIC RECOGNITION BY AMERICAN MEDICAL PHYSICIANS

Nielsen, J. M., M.D., *Clinical Neurology*, Paul B. Hoeber, Inc., N.Y., 1946.
Lewin, Philip, M.D., *The Back and Its Disc Syndrome*, Lea and Febiger, 1955.
"Neck is Cause of Headaches, Study Hints," *Chicago Tribune*, May 7, 1970.
Pottenger, F. M., *Symptoms of Visceral Disease*, Mosby, St. Louis, Missouri, 1953.
The ACA Journal of Chiropractic, November 1969, page 7 (Ruegseggar treating trigger points).
Wright, Jessie, M.D., "Mechanics in Relation to Derangements of the Facet Joints of the Spine," *Archives of Physical Therapy*, April 1944, pages 201–206.
Hadley, Lee, M.D., "Intervertebral Joint Subluxation, Bony Impingement and Foramen Encroachment with Nerve Root Changes," *American Journal of Roentgenology*, Vol. 65, 1951, pages 377–401.
Mennell, John M., *Back Pain*, Little Brown, Boston, 1960.
Park, Richard, B.S.; Tapp, Jessie, M.D.; Hochstrasser, D. L., Ph.D.,

"Chiropractors and Patients in Kentucky," *Journal of the Kentucky Medical Association*, Vol. 65, No. 11, November 1967, pages 1101–1104.
"Sciatica," *Merck Manual*, Merck and Company, Inc., Rahway, N.J., Eighth Edition, 1950, page 1029.
"Headaches," *Merck Manual*, Merck and Company, Inc., Rahway, N.J., 11th Edition, 1966, page 998.
Baum, Allyn Z., "Who on Earth Goes to a Chiropractor?" (from the *Congressional Record*, Washington, June 16, 1972).

Chapter 16. CHIROPRACTIC RECOGNITION IN OTHER COUNTRIES

Germany

C. W. Weiant, D.C., Ph.D., and S. Goldschmidt, D.C., "What Medicine Really Thinks About Chiropractic," American Chiropractic Association, Des Moines, Iowa, 1966 (various references to Drs. Zukschwerdt, Rocher, Cramer, Gutmann, Kusche, Kemlin, Hochfeld, Boje).
Biederman, Freimut, M.D., "Fundamentals of Chiropractic from the Standpoint of a Medical Doctor," ICRC—Davenport, Iowa, 1959 (English translation by L. C. J. Iekeler, D.C.).
G. Gutmann, M.D., *Hippokrates*, September 15, 1957, page 539 (high costs superfluous if chiropractic was applied).

Russia

Speransky, A.D., *A Basis for the Theory of Medicine*, Director of the Department of Pathophysiology of the All Union Institute of Experimental Medicine, Leningrad, International Publishers, N.Y., 1943.

England

Mennell, James, M.D., *The Science and Art of Joint Manipulation*, Vol. 2, The Spinal Column, J. and A. Churchill, London, 1952.
"Spinal Manipulation for Back Pain Urged," *Los Angeles Times*, March 14, 1971 (James Henry Cyriax lecture at the California Medical Association).
"Should MDs Manipulate Backs?" Focus on the News, *Medical World News*, McGraw-Hill Publication, April 2, 1971, Vol. 12, No. 20, page 4 (comments on James Henry Cyriax).
"Backache Cure," Parade section, *Chicago Sun-Times*, December 19, 1971 (reference to James Henry Cyriax).
Bourdillon, J. F., M.D., *Spinal Manipulation*, Appleton-Century-Crofts, Meredith Corporation, N.Y., 1970 (an unbiased assessment of chiropractic needed, page 9; reference to deafness, page 131).

Canada

"Chiropractic Profession Welcomes Views of Quebec Royal Commission," *Journal of the Canadian Chiropractic Association*, December–January 1965–1966, page 7.

"A Report on the Findings of the Lacroix Commission in the Province of Quebec," *Journal of the Canadian Chiropractic Association*, December–January 1965–1966, pages 8–12.

"CMA Amends Code of Ethics—Encourages Cooperation," *Journal of the Canadian Chiropractic Association*, March 1971, page 5.

Toronto Globe and Mail, February 13, 1971 (no longer unethical for MDs to refer to chiropractors in Canada).

Parsons, W. B., M.D., *Canadian Medical Journal*, July 15, 1958.

Denmark, Austria, Australia

Bøze, *Ugeskrift for Laeger*, August 30, 1956.

France

McClusky, Thorp, *Your Health and Chiropractic*, Pyramid Books, N.Y., 1962 (reference to Adolph Lorenz, M.D.).

Japan

"60 Japanese Doctors Visit N.C.C.," *News Bulletin*, National College of Chiropractic, Lombard, Illinois, July 1971.

Chapter 17. RESEARCH SUPPORTS CHIROPRACTIC

Nordstrom, B. E., D.C., "Bioengineering Analysis of Spinal Systems," Public Information Director, International Chiropractors Association, Davenport, Iowa, October 22, 1971 (Bioengineering Analysis of Spinal Systems).

"A Clinical Study of the Low Back Factors," American Chiropractic Association, Des Moines, Iowa, 1972 (Rensselaer Polytechnic Institute project).

"Nixon Signs Bill Providing $2 million for Chiropractic Research." International Chiropractors Association, Davenport, Iowa, December 21, 1973.

Institute for the Study of the Mechanics, Statics and Dynamics of the Human Body

Illi, F. W. *Kurzer* Abriss der Chiropraktik, Geneva, 1933; *Die Wahrheit* uber die Chiropraktik, Geneva, 1938; *Medicine ou Chiropratique*—Association des Chiropracticiens, Suisses, Berne, 1939.

Medizin, Uberflug and Chiropraktik—Geneva, 1950; *The Vertebral Column,*

Life-Line of the Body, Chicago, 1951; *Chiropratique, Locomotion, Statique Vertebrale*, Geneva, 1952 (above information compiled and catalogued by Illi)

Nerve Compression and Disease

Haldeman, Scott and Meyer, B. J., "The Effect of Experimental Constriction on the Structure of the Sciatic Nerve," *South African Journal of Laboratory and Clinical Medicine*, August 8, 1970, pages 888–892.

Haldeman, Scott and Drum, D., "The Compression Subluxation," The Journal of *Clinical Chiropractic—Archives No. 1*, Spring 1971 (reference to Haldeman, Gelfan and Tarlov (1956), Bentley and Schlapp, Causey and Palmer, Weiss and Hiscoe (1969), Causey and Werner (1950), Droz and Leblond (1962), von Breeman et al., (1958), Hebb and Silver (1961).

Haldeman, Scott and Meyer, B. J., "The Effect of Constriction of the Action Potential in the Sciatic Nerve," *South African Journal of Laboratory and Clinical Medicine*, August 8, 1970, pages 903–906.

Cole, W. V., D.O., "The Osteopathic Lesion Complex—The Effects of the Experimental Osteopathic Lesion, Chemical Irritants in the Muscle at the Level of the Sixth Thoracic Segment, and Chemical Irritants in the Liver," *Journal of the American Osteopathic Association*, November 1949.

Cole, W. V., D.O., "Somaticovisceral Reflexes—A Preliminary Report of the Experimental Aspect of Somaticovisceral Reflexes Immediately Following Electrical Stimulation and a Minor Vertebral Strain," *Journal of the American Osteopathic Association*, May 1951.

Cole, W. V., D.O., "Somaticovisceral Reflexes—The Effects of Spinal Fixation at the Thoracolumbar Junction on Certain Visceral Structures," *Journal of the American Osteopathic Association*, February 1953.

Department of Research and Statistics

Higley, Henry, M.S., D.C., "The Intervertebral Disc Syndrome," Research Report, National Chiropractic Association, Webster City, Iowa, January 1960 (now the ACA, Des Moines, Iowa).

Other Research Projects

Dintenfass, Julius, D.C., *Chiropractic, A Modern Way to Health*, Pyramid Books, N.Y., 1970 (quoting from *Journal of Clinical Chiropractic*, N.Y., Vol. 1, No. 4).

Quigley, W.H., D.C. and Pullella, Santo, Ph.D., Palmer College of Chiropractic, Davenport, Iowa (clinical studies of effects of exercise upon patients).

Conclusion

"Chiropractic Survey and Statistical Study," Batten and Associates, Management Consultants, Des Moines, Iowa, 1963, page 38, No. 82 (chiropractic profession supports research shown on poll).

Chapter 18. PROMINENT PEOPLE SUPPORT CHIROPRACTIC

Parker, James, *The Teach-In News*, Share International, 1970, Vol. 1, No. 1, pages 1–8 (reference to prominent people supporting chiropractic).
"The Chiropractic Documentary Movie," *The Digest of Chiropractic Economics*, November 1972 (interview with the director, Mr. Patrick McGoohan).
Sordoni, Andrew, "Chiropractic in Industry," American Chiropractic Association, Des Moines, Iowa, August 17, 1965.
"Who Really Helped Her to Walk Again?" *Healthways Magazine*, American Chiropractic Association, Des Moines, Iowa, December 1956, Vol. 11, No. 7 (story of a March of Dimes Polio "Model").
Robertson, Lewis, *Manual of Acute and Chronic Poliomyelitis*, Polio Foundation of California, Santa Cruz, California, 1955, pages 50–51 (reference to Winifred Gardella with pictures and notorized statement).
Wilson, E. G., Notary Public for Santa Cruz County, Commission expired November 26, 1958 (statement by Mrs. Joseph Gardella, paternal grandmother).
"Hubert Humphrey's Chiropractor Flown to California to Give Veep Adjustment," *Journal of the American Chiropractic Association*, September 9, 1968.

Index

NOTES

NOTES

NOTES

NOTES